A
PHYSICIAN
in the AGE
of LIBERAL
REFORM

NEW **HISPANISMS**
Cultural and Literary Studies

ANNE J. CRUZ, SERIES EDITOR

A

PHYSICIAN

in the AGE

of LIBERAL

REFORM

ILDEFONSO MARTÍNEZ Y FERNÁNDEZ

and MEDICAL POLITICS *in*

NINETEENTH-CENTURY SPAIN

A N D R E W   W.   K E I T T

LOUISIANA STATE UNIVERSITY PRESS
Baton Rouge

Published by Louisiana State University Press
lsupress.org

Designer: Kaelin Chappell Broaddus
Typefaces: Adobe Caslon Pro, text; Antiquarian Scribe, Old Kirk WF, and Pomeroy WF, display

Portions of chapter 4, "Medical Martyrs," first appeared as "Medical Martyrs:
Nineteenth-Century Representations of Early Modern Inquisitorial Persecution of
Spanish Physicians" in *Early Science and Medicine* 23 (January 2018): 135–158.

Cataloging-in-Publication Data are available at the Library of Congress.

ISBN 978-0-8071-8228-4 (cloth) | ISBN 978-0-8071-8317-5 (pdf) |
ISBN 978-0-8071-8316-8 (epub)

This book is dedicated to my mother,

Ruth Gouverneur Morris Keitt

(APRIL 9, 1937–OCTOBER 27, 2020),

and to all the health-care professionals
who put their lives at risk treating
the victims of the COVID-19 pandemic.

Contents

Preface

In the spring of 2016 I received an invitation to contribute to a special issue of the journal *Early Science and Medicine* on medicine and the Inquisition. While I had written previously on medicine and the Spanish Inquisition in the sixteenth and seventeenth centuries, I had since moved on to other topics, but the project description sounded intriguing, and with a research trip to Spain on the horizon I asked for some time to explore the possibilities. Upon arriving at the National Library in Madrid, I embarked on a cursory search of the catalog and, as fate would have it, the first document to appear was a nineteenth-century work entitled "Physicians Persecuted by the Spanish Inquisition" by Ildefonso Martínez y Fernández. Martínez was a physician and liberal reformer whose collected papers, in another fortuitous coincidence, had recently been cataloged across town at the Marqués de Valdecilla Historical Library of the Complutense University of Madrid.[1]

Although I had not envisioned undertaking a project dealing with nineteenth-century Spain, I found myself fascinated by Martínez's writings, which touched on physiology, epidemiology, mental illness, philosophy, literature, history, politics, and many other topics. As it turned out, Martínez's intellectual project was related to work I had previously done on medicine and politics in early modern Spain.[2] In fact, Martínez was an expositor of an important early modern medico-political corpus epitomized by works such as *La nueva filosofía de la naturaleza del hombre* (*The New Philosophy of Human Nature*), by Oliva Sabuco de Nantes Barrera, and *El examen de ingenios* (*The Examination of Men's Wits*) by Juan Huarte de San Juan—both of which Martínez reedited in the mid-nineteenth century.

Ildefonso Martínez lived during a period beset by political turmoil and pandemic disease; he was born in 1821 in the aftermath of a military uprising and died of cholera in 1855 in the wake of a popular revolution. The period was also characterized by the consolidation of a new, liberal regime and the renovation of the medical profession after a series of sociopolitical upheavals in the first two decades of the century. These two historical phenomena were not unrelated, as physicians played important roles in liberal politics during the period, both as actual politicians and as contributors to a new political culture. It was in this latter capacity that Martínez operated when he wrote his treatise on physicians who ran afoul of the Inquisition, a work that was by no means a dispassionate exercise in the history of medicine, but rather a broadside against Church and Crown in the old regime, two of Spanish liberals' favorite targets.

This book explores, among other things, the "uses of the past" by Spanish liberals in general and Ildefonso Martínez in particular. Martínez and his peers reenvisioned the history of Spain to serve their own contemporary political agenda—they held a mirror up to the past, but at an angle that reflected what they wanted to see. What I could not have imagined when beginning this project was how the themes it deals with would come to be reflected in our present moment. In 2016, political insurrections and pandemics seemed to be scourges that conveniently afflicted other times and places, but on January 6, 2021, during the bicentennial year of Martínez's birth, the United States witnessed an attempted insurrection which sought to block the peaceful transfer of power for the first time in the nation's history, and this unprecedented attack on American democracy took place in the midst of a global pandemic, which as of this writing has killed approximately seven million worldwide, including beloved members of my own family.

Thus, this book, by necessity, grapples with the issue of how the present comes to be interpreted through the prism of the past, and by the same token, how the past is interpreted in light of the preoccupations of the present. Events from the period in which Ildefonso Martínez lived have come to resonate with contemporary events in ways that could not have been predicted, and they have now taken on a tragic relevance. So, at the risk of relying excessively on optical metaphors, during the writing of this book I have sometimes had the strange sensation of inhabiting a historical hall of mirrors. It is, of course, the job of a historian to clarify our perspectives on the past, despite our inevitable historical situatedness, and to provide insight into the ways in which historical narratives both enlighten and obscure. I will let my readers judge whether I have succeeded in this task.

Acknowledgments

This book began with an invitation, so I want to thank Maria Pia Donato at the outset. It was Maria Pia's invitation to contribute to her edited volume on medicine and the Inquisition that initiated this project and sent me to the archives in search of material. My serendipitous encounter with the work of Ildefonso Martínez y Fernández was facilitated by librarian Eduardo Anglada Monzón. As it happened, the first document by Martínez that I discovered was written under a pseudonym, and Eduardo assisted me in ferreting out the true identity of the author. With this information in hand, I paid a visit to Mercedes Cabello Martín, archivist at the Historical Library of the Complutense University. Mercedes would go on to support the research for this book in a variety ways, and for that I am deeply grateful.

Any book is inevitably a collective effort, but in this case it is especially true. Because this book represents something of a departure from my previous work, I benefited greatly from the advice of a number of scholars who were exceptionally generous with their expertise. Three people in particular merit special recognition: Elizabeth Williams shared a long and illustrious career's worth of knowledge concerning the history of nineteenth-century medicine and guided my initial explorations into the "science of man"; Jon Arrizabalaga provided unfailing support and inspiration throughout my research and writing with recommendations of many things to read and people to contact; Enric Novella fielded an out-of-the-blue email from a stranger and responded with both erudition and hospitality, providing not only scholarly insight, but also a memorable tour of his hometown of Valencia. All three read the entire manuscript and offered invaluable suggestions for improvement. A host of others graciously entertained my importunate entreaties, including Rafael Huertas, Mario César Sánchez Villa, Luis Montiel, Víctor Álvarez Antuña, and Juan Sisinio Pérez Garzón. I want to thank Jaime

Elipe for tracking down one last cache of documents in the archives for me, and Ismael del Olmo for reading the manuscript and for his contributions to the scholarship on Juan Huarte. I am grateful to the staff of Marcial Pons bookstore in Madrid, who over the years have never failed to recommend key secondary sources for whatever project I happened to be working on. Thanks go to John Moore and Brian Steele, who were fellow members of a writing group that witnessed the process up close and personal. I wish to acknowledge Richard Herr, who long ago kindled my interest in Spanish history and who passed away as this book was nearing completion. As always, I am deeply indebted to my doctoral advisor, Randy Starn, who after all these many years continues to be an inspiration. I only hope that I can become as good a mentor to my students as he has been to me. Ultimately, the intellectual debts I have incurred in writing this book are too numerous to fully list here, but I am truly thankful for all the gifts I have received and recognize that they made the finished product much better than it would have otherwise been. Of course, the inevitable errors and oversights remain mine alone.

I also received crucial institutional support while pursuing this project. First and foremost, the Department of History at the University of Alabama at Birmingham provided a collegial atmosphere as well as more tangible forms of support. Chair Jonathan Wiesen and staff members Jerrie McCurry and Robin Albarano deserve special thanks for their dedication to making the department such a hospitable place to research and teach. Graduate students Christian Stockdill, Jacob Kennedy, and Kamau Davis did yeoman's work helping me dot the i's and cross the t's. A shout-out to Filter Coffee Parlor for allowing me to monopolize the corner table next to the wall outlet. The College of Arts and Sciences at UAB provided several research grants that made it possible to travel to Spain to conduct the archival research that forms the basis of this book. I thank the staff at UAB's Mervyn Sterne Library, and especially Eddie Luster in Interlibrary Loan. The Association for Spanish and Portuguese Historical Studies and the European Section of the Southern Historical Society provided forums for presenting my research in progress, which in turn afforded opportunities to gain valuable feedback. Thanks to Brill Academic Publishers for granting permission to use previously published material. I am grateful to Stan Ivester for his meticulous copy editing, and to the anonymous readers who reviewed the manuscript for Louisiana State University Press. Finally, I offer special thanks to James Long and Anne Cruz for believing in this project at a very early stage, and for their considerable efforts in shepherding it to completion.

Pandemic amnesia seems to be an inevitable response in the wake of widespread contagions of infectious disease, and so it may well be the case that, as you are reading this, the COVID-19 pandemic appears as a vague fever dream from the distant past. Please let me assure you that in the spring of 2020 it was all too real, especially for health-care workers who were reading reports of their colleagues dying while caring for COVID patients. While I was safely ensconced behind the computer keyboard, my wife, Aileen, was on the front lines as a dental hygienist in those early days, and her professionalism, courage, and dedication to her patients were an inspiration. Her knowledge of infection control and conscientiousness about masking kept our household safe during the period before the advent of COVID vaccines. Other members of our family were not so fortunate. In the fall of 2020, COVID swept through the assisted-living facility where my mother, Ruth, was living. She contracted the virus and died on October 27 of that year.

My mother was a remarkable person who never took the predictable path, and she, together with my father, created a home that was encouraging of creativity and conducive to the love of ideas. I credit them both with nurturing my curiosity about the world and thank them for never questioning my determination to craft a career dedicated to thinking and writing. Yet, such a career presents its own set of challenges for one's loved ones, who stand by, year after year, as a manuscript gradually takes shape. I am grateful to Aileen for her patience, and to our son, Seaver, who has been watching this project progress for half his lifetime. Additionally, I want to express my appreciation to my in-laws, Bellie and Roger Guerrero, who generously helped with child-care on many occasions while I was working in the archives.

In the summer of 2022 I traveled to Oviedo, in the north of Spain, in order to examine documents concerning the circumstances surrounding the death of Ildefonso Martínez y Fernández. In an ironic twist of fate, this trip to conduct research on a nineteenth-century pandemic had been repeatedly delayed due to a twenty-first-century pandemic, which had made international travel difficult if not impossible. I must admit, however, that my motives for the journey were not entirely scholarly; I felt personally drawn to the site of Martínez's death, having spent the previous six years immersed in his life story.

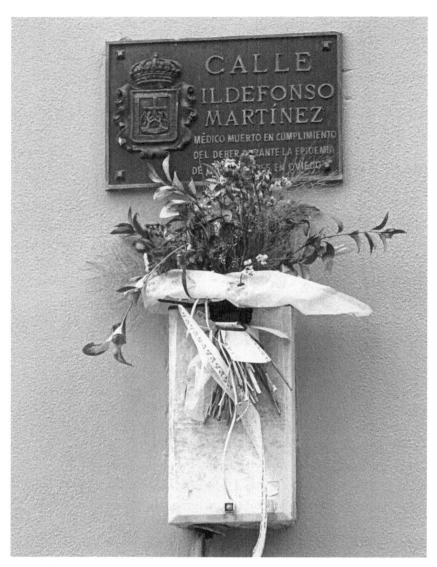

Plaque dedicated to Ildefonso Martínez, "a physician who died while doing his duty during the cholera epidemic of 1855 in Oviedo." Author's photograph.

One of the landmarks I was particularly eager to visit was a street that had been renamed in his honor. As it turned out, calle Ildefonso Martínez was a graffiti-strewn alleyway, home to the Salsipuedes DiscoBar ("Salsipuedes" being the former name of the street). Undeterred by this unprepossessing vista, I wandered to the far end of the alley, where I found a plaque in honor of Martínez, and to my great surprise, a bouquet of flowers underneath, which had been placed there by a neighborhood organization in his memory. Apparently, I was not the only one to have taken an interest in Martínez, or to have made the connection between the 1855 cholera outbreak and the current COVID-19 pandemic.

I spent the next several days in the Municipal Archive of Oviedo, engrossed in accounts of the cholera pandemic, reading about hospitals being overwhelmed and bodies piling up in the streets. Then I took the train back to Madrid and the following day tested positive for COVID-19, having somehow managed to avoid the virus over the previous two and a half years. Of course, by the summer of 2022 a COVID infection in someone who had been vaccinated was a minor inconvenience, a far cry from a deadly bout of cholera, but nevertheless it seemed an uncanny scenario to have contracted an infectious disease in the city where the subject of my research died of one. I take this episode as one final example of how the life of Ildefonso Martínez y Fernández has resonated into the present.

A
PHYSICIAN
in the AGE
of LIBERAL
REFORM

Introduction
Revolutionizing *la Medicina Patria*

Spanish physicians were a political force in the nineteenth century during the tumultuous process of nation-building that followed the War of Independence against the Napoleonic invasion of the Iberian peninsula (1808–14). Many participated in the Cortes of Cádiz, which in 1812 drafted Spain's first constitution, and went on to play important roles in the public sphere and in the legislature during the "liberal revolution," which undertook the establishment of a new, and precarious, liberal order. This book deals with the life and work of one such physician: Ildefonso Martínez y Fernández, whose brief career coincided with the consolidation of the liberal revolution and the drive to reform and professionalize Spanish medicine, or *la medicina patria*. Born in 1821, Martínez was not only a physician, but also a polymath and political activist whose prolific literary and scholarly output made him a fixture in the political and intellectual ferment of mid-nineteenth-century Spain, until his untimely death in the cholera epidemic of 1854–55. Martínez is an important, yet neglected, figure in the history of Spanish medicine, one who produced a significant body of intellectual work, made key contributions to the profession, and cultivated a deep engagement with the political struggles of the period.[1]

The relationship between medicine and politics, however, was not limited to the efforts of medical professionals to navigate the new political realities of the emerging liberal regime; while physicians such as Ildefonso Martínez were politically active during this period, medicine itself had taken on an increasingly political dimension. In the second half of the eighteenth century, a transformation occurred in European ideas concerning the role of medicine in society, a transformation which gave rise to an anthropological notion of medicine as an all-encompassing "science of man" that would govern the health not only of individual bodies, but of the body politic as well. The science of man is often associated with the Revolutionary period in France, but its origins predate the French Revolution, and its legacy extends well beyond, both temporally and geographically.[2]

The science of man exerted a powerful influence in nineteenth-century Spain, as has been amply documented by Spanish scholars.[3] What has been less than fully appreciated is the continued influence in Spain of an early modern medico-political discourse that anticipated the science of man. There arose in the sixteenth century a "medical humanism" which flourished as a movement dedicated not only to the discovery and translation of ancient medical works, but also to the development of a medical politics geared toward social and political reform—a science of man *avant la lettre*.[4] Two of the crowning glories of this tradition in Spain were *La nueva filosofía de la naturaleza del hombre* by Oliva Sabuco de Nantes Barrera and *El examen de ingenios para las ciencias* by Juan Huarte de San Juan. Not only did Martínez produce new editions of these works, he also commented extensively on them in annotations to the texts themselves, in articles published in the medical press, and in presentations given to professional societies. Remarkably, despite a plethora of secondary literature on Sabuco and Huarte, there has been virtually nothing written on their influence in the nineteenth century, and their chief expositor, Ildefonso Martínez y Fernández, has suffered a similar neglect.[5] This book seeks to fill these lacunae, and in the process show how Martínez's engagement with these classic works was not a mere exercise in antiquarianism, but rather a project aimed at deploying them in contemporary medico-political debates. The science of man sought to harmonize "the physical and moral aspects of man," and in so doing kindled debates on topics ranging from the mind-body problem, to the relationship between religious truth and political legitimacy, to the nature of race and gender.

While Ildefonso Martínez's attempts to link key works in the history of Spanish medicine with the science of man are an important part of the story, they must be seen in the wider context of a new liberal political culture that was emerging in nineteenth-century Spain. Liberal intellectuals like Martínez were both products and producers of this political culture, and as is so often the case, creative "uses of the past" figured prominently in this recursive process. Martínez and his peers appropriated the history of Spain for the purposes of their own nineteenth-century political project, and this of course was nothing new; just as Martínez's forays into the history of medicine were shaped by his nineteenth-century political agenda, the Renaissance sources he selectively appropriated were themselves, in turn, based on selective appropriations of classical antiquity, and so on and so forth.[6]

So this is a biography of a nineteenth-century Spanish physician, and as such it combines three elements that have given rise to countless controversies: biography, nineteenth-century Spain, and the history of Spanish medicine and science. With this in mind, before further detailing what this book is about, I want to pause in order to explain what it is *not* about.

This is not a book about the relative merit of Spain's medical and scientific achievements. Debates over Spain's contributions to European science have been dubbed the "polemic of Spanish science," and this was for many years the defining discourse in the history of science pertaining to Spain. The polemic was initiated in 1782 by the French *philosophe* Nicolas Masson de Morvilliers, who posed the question with regard to scientific progress, "What do we owe to Spain?" For Morvilliers, the question was rhetorical, and the answer was, "nothing at all"; Spain's intrinsic superstition and fanatical religiosity, buttressed by a tyrannical Inquisition, made scientific progress impossible.[7] Morvilliers's provocation congealed into conventional wisdom among many scholars outside Spain and set in motion an incessant back-and-forth among Spanish historians of science, some of whom put forward a patriotic defense of Iberian science against its detractors, while others echoed the assessment of Spain's critics, often with a political agenda of their own aimed at implicating the ruling class in what they perceived to be the country's failure to modernize.[8] In either case, Spain was viewed as exceptional, possessed of a unique national character that could explain, on the one hand, the calumnies launched against her achievements by jealous partisans, or on the other, the inability of Spain to keep pace with her European neighbors.

The polemic on Spanish science has cast a long shadow, as Juan Pimentel and José Pardo-Tomás have observed.[9] Even in the work of serious scholars who have made important contributions to Spanish history of science, there have often been implicit comparisons with a master narrative of European modernization, and the Scientific Revolution is smuggled in the back door, albeit in a "problematized" form. So we get historical accounts that portray

Spain as a scientific innovator on par with other European nations, but in the context of a broadened Scientific Revolution that valorizes the practical sciences as equal to the theoretical ones. In such accounts, much emphasis is given to Spanish medicine, which in the sixteenth century championed post-Vesalian anatomy, often considered to be a harbinger of the Scientific Revolution, and in the late seventeenth century gave birth to the reform movement, or *movimiento novator*, which denounced the regnant Galenism of the medical establishment and advocated for novel theories such as the circulation of the blood, thereby positioning itself at the cutting edge of scientific innovation.[10] Pimentel and Pardo-Tomás point to the canonical collection of essays *Beyond the Black Legend: Spain and the Scientific Revolution* as another example of the subtle reach of the polemic, noting that many of the essays reproduce arguments from the polemic even while attempting to distance themselves from them.[11] Pimentel and Pardo-Tomás suggest that this perceived need to mainstream the history of Spanish science was in keeping with a more generalized desire to situate Spain within the prevailing narrative of European modernity during Spain's transition to democracy in the post-Franco era.

In closing, Pimentel and Pardo-Tomás highlight the irony of attempts to align Spanish science with a process of modernization epitomized by the Scientific Revolution, given that the very concept of a unitary "modernity" has been undermined in recent years—in the work of Bruno Latour, for example.[12] For Pimentel and Pardo-Tomás, a "heterogeneous" and "kaleidoscopic" conception of modernity may not only be more accurate, but also more propitious for understanding the relationship between science and the Iberian world. With these caveats in mind, I have no intention of revisiting old arguments surrounding the status of Spanish science and medicine; instead, I will limit my focus to medical discourse in the context of the consolidation of the liberal revolution in Spain.

Moving on to the political history of nineteenth-century Spain, this is not a book about the "dysfunction" of Spanish politics, or the inability of Spaniards to hew to an arbitrary metric of national development.[13] As with Spanish science, Spanish politics has typically been judged and found wanting according to an idealized standard. Exhibit A in this litigation is the familiar pattern that began during the liberal revolution of the nineteenth century in which fragile governing structures were at the mercy of reactionary forces, whether in the form of monarchist uprisings or military *pronunciamientos*. Although there is no denying the turbulence of Spain's nineteenth-century political history, accounts of this history have all too often taken the form of a morality tale, rife with "stereotyping, simplification, and Manicheanism," as Stanley Payne has duly noted.[14] In this tale, the standard that Spain inevitably failed to live up to was the Anglo-American political tradition, which saw itself as "republican, entrepreneurial, rational," while Spain was inherently "monarchist, indolent, fanatical."[15] This "juxtaposition of Spanish decadence and Anglo-American progress" has been dubbed "Prescott's paradigm" by Richard Kagan, in reference to William H. Prescott, the Harvard-educated historian who was one of the earliest and most influential scholars to introduce these tropes into the historiography of Spain.[16]

Prescott's paradigm is a good example of how historiographic frameworks are often forged on the anvil of contemporary concerns; it was a cautionary tale in which Spain functioned as a foil for America's exceptionalist self-image. As Edward Peters has pointed out, early nineteenth-century Romantic historians like Prescott perceived national unity to be the key political achievement of the modern world. They saw Spain's early history, from the medieval period through the reign of Isabel and Fernando, as an example of successful state building, and as a positive model for the United States, both countries having weathered similar internecine struggles on the road to establishing a strong central government and having had to deal with "decadent," "barbaric" peoples in their midst—the Jews and Muslims in the case of Spain, and indigenous peoples in the American case.[17] Both governments were seen as having consolidated sovereignty while respecting democratic traditions and regional autonomy, but with the arrival of the "despotism" imposed by the Habsburg monarchs in league with the Catholic Church, Spanish political history parted ways with the American exemplar. Prescott's paradigm has had a long-lasting influence, and although historians have persistently chipped away at popular, oversimplified notions of Spanish decline and decadence, as Kagan writes, "America's identity may still depend on national histories that are both conceived and constructed as antithetical to its own."[18]

But a funny thing happened during the writing of this book. The very same Anglo-American political tradition that has so often been held up as a yardstick to measure Spain's perceived failures began to exhibit weaknesses of its own. On June 23, 2016, only weeks after I began my research, the United

Kingdom voted to leave the European Union in what was widely seen as a portent of a global retreat from the cosmopolitan liberal order in favor of a populist nationalism. Then, on November 8 of that same year, the American people elected Donald J. Trump as president, and in so doing set the stage for an unprecedented assault on the foundations of liberal democracy in the United States. On January 6, 2021, in the wake of Donald Trump's electoral defeat, supporters of the ex-president stormed the Capitol seeking to block the counting of Electoral College ballots, and thereby disrupt the peaceful transfer of power for the first time in the nation's history. While the attempted insurrection was unsuccessful, it should stand as a warning to those who would posit an innate Anglo-American aptitude for self-governance and liberal democracy.

Given these recent events, it seems the time has come to lay aside the last vestiges of Prescott's paradigm once and for all, and with them the shopworn essentialism that has all too often characterized the writing of Spanish history. In laying to rest a framework that has engendered too many facile contrasts and oversimplifications, we may come to see Spain as "one more variant of a richly diverse European story."[19] Indeed, when it comes to studying the history of nineteenth-century Spain, a new generation of historians has emerged, intent on reinterpreting the history of Spanish liberalism in a more nuanced fashion.[20] These historians have shown that the liberal revolution was "a phenomenon much richer, more vital, and more diverse, than previously thought."[21] I conceive of the present work as part of this historiographic project.

Turning now from a discussion of content to a discussion of form, this book centers on a particular life, which brings us to the third area of contention: biography as a genre and methodology. This book is *not* a traditional biography. Traditional biography as a form of historical scholarship dedicated to chronicling the exploits of "great men" has been much maligned—and not without reason; from the partisans of the *Annales* school with their emphasis on deep-seated social structures and collective *mentalités,* to postmodernist theorists heralding the "death of the subject," traditional biography was often portrayed as an outmoded approach with little to contribute in terms of methodological rigor or theoretical sophistication.[22] In Spain biography has been doubly suspect, given its prominent role in lionizing heroes of the Franco regime.[23] Over the past several decades, however, scholars have availed themselves of new biographical approaches that have moved beyond hagiography toward forms of historical biography that bring to bear insights from social and cultural history, and in so doing highlight complex relationships between the individual and the collective.[24]

Interestingly, the history of nineteenth-century Spain has been one of the foremost avenues for this biographical turn, due in in no small measure to the efforts of Isabel Burdiel, who is not only one of the foremost historians of nineteenth-century Spain, but also a pioneer of the new historical biography. For Burdiel, the individual life no longer functions as an ideal type asserted to be representative of a larger group, or as a lens that magically brings into focus the "spirit of the age," but rather as a space in which a variety of methodologies and potential frames of analysis can coexist in creative tension.[25]

One methodology that Burdiel invokes is microhistory—she quotes approvingly the microhistorical dictum that, while the questions historians address should be general, and even universal, the answers should be local and particular.[26] Burdiel is not alone in advocating a cross-fertilization between microhistory and historical biography; such an approach has also been advocated by the Dutch School of biographical studies represented by scholars such as Hans Renders and Binne de Haan.[27] The present study is to some extent microhistorical, drawing as it does on fragmentary source materials pertaining to a relatively obscure figure. We have very little in the way of precise biographical details when it comes to Ildefonso Martínez y Fernández. We are not privy to the details of his medical practice, or the nature of his religious affiliation (or lack thereof), and we have no information concerning his personal relationships. What we do have are his collected papers, his writings—and writings about him—in the periodical press, and his copious annotations to the works he edited. These resources provide more than enough material to explore, as Giovanni Levi urged historians to do, "the links that tie together a social field and an acting person."[28]

Just as a reinvigorated genre of historical biography has helped illuminate the history of nineteenth-century Spain, biography has enjoyed a similar renaissance in the history of science and medicine over the past thirty years.[29] Once shunned as a vestige of an outdated heroic history of science, biography has moved from chronicling the solitary exploits of scientific "geniuses" to a more balanced treatment of individual lives contextualized within larger structures. Thus, Steven Shapin's work on Robert Boyle becomes a meditation on the changing social role of the natural philosopher in early modern Europe, while Roy Porter's biography of Thomas Beddoes seeks to shed light on "the sickness culture of late-Enlightenment England."[30] The esteemed historian of medicine Charles Rosenberg has argued that a revised conceptualization of biography "constitutes an indispensable tool for the collective historical enterprise," insofar as "a life can be construed as a sampling device—as a controlled and internally coherent batch of data, a chronologically ordered set of realities and relationships perceived and understood by a particular actor."[31]

What this book *is* about is how the "realities and relationships" at work in the life of Ildefonso Martínez intersected with numerous aspects of mid-nineteenth-century Spanish society and culture, given his various roles as a medical student and physician, as an advocate for, and critic of, the medical profession, as a journalist and political polemicist, and as a medical historian and man of letters. My goal is not to argue that Martínez was somehow exemplary of Spanish physicians as a whole, or that he exercised a hitherto unappreciated influence on the development of Spanish medicine, but rather that his life can help illuminate the various roles played by both medical practitioners and medical discourse during the Spanish liberal revolution of the nineteenth century.

But what, precisely, do we mean when speaking of the "liberal revolution?" This is not an easy question to answer for a number of reasons, the first of which being that the word "liberal" is notoriously polysemic and was in a state of flux during precisely the period under study here. In its adjectival form, the term was widely used in England and France during the eighteenth century to describe ideas and opinions related to constitutionalism, limited government, and individual rights. It was in Spain, however, in the early nineteenth century, that the adjective "liberal" gave way to the substantive forms, "liberalism" and "liberal," which came to denote a revolutionary commitment to political liberty and to describe a member of a political party dedicated to such a proposition.[32] This etymological association between liberalism and revolution was due in large part to the efforts of Spanish insurgents during the War of Independence, as they sought to frame their struggle against absolute monarchy and foreign occupation in terms of liberal principles such as freedom of the press, equality before the law, the expansion of voting rights, and the loosening of old-regime economic restrictions.[33]

In addition to these linguistic complexities, the situation is complicated further still by political schisms within Spanish liberalism itself. An example of such a schism occurred during what came to be known as the Liberal Triennium (1820–23), when a liberal government briefly ruled after a military uprising overthrew the restored Bourbon monarchy of Fernando VII. It was at this time that the Spanish liberal coalition fragmented and ultimately bifurcated into factions which vied against each other as putative heirs to the true liberal tradition. These two factions, the *moderados* and *exaltados,* initiated a rift that would come to characterize Spanish liberalism throughout the nineteenth century. On the one hand, the moderados argued that the achievements of the liberal revolution should be consolidated under a constitutional monarchy that would maintain order and safeguard private property. On the other hand, the exaltados insisted that the gains of the revolution had to be extended more broadly, and the last vestiges of the old regime brought to heel, even if that entailed social unrest and political upheaval. Thus, the Spanish liberal revolution came to comprise a wide ideological spectrum that included both radical republicans and "moderate" constitutional monarchists, who, paradoxically, took positions that were not particularly revolutionary, and in fact could often be quite conservative.

Given the complexities of the Spanish liberal revolution, how can we best summarize its essential components and articulate its role in the present study? In the broadest sense, the effect of the liberal revolution, according to Isabel Burdiel, was to "forge a new political arrangement of the mechanisms of social and economic power, and of the sources of cultural legitimacy, which had already undergone substantial change during the eighteenth century. The importance of those earlier changes, together with the impact of the crisis initiated by the Napoleonic invasion in 1808, is what defines the specific character of what contemporaries called 'the Spanish revolution.'"[34] The focus of this book is the role of medicine as a discourse, and as a profession, in the construction of the "mechanisms of social and economic power" and the "sources of cultural legitimacy" mentioned by Burdiel. Revolutionizing la medicina patria, then, was the process through which Spanish medicine sought to assert itself in a new social and economic order and participate in the formation of a new political culture for liberal Spain. This process was carried out not only in the legislature, in which numerous physicians served, but also in countless treatises advocating a prominent role for medicine in governing the body politic.[35] In Spain, as elsewhere, physicians were influential public intellectuals who portrayed medicine as a "useful profession" that could benefit the emerging liberal state. Ildefonso Martínez played an important role in this process, one that has been overlooked.

The concept of "political culture" merits some clarification. In the most basic sense, a political culture can be defined as "a conjunction of representations that configure a human group in political terms, which is to say, a shared vision of the world, a common reading of history, an imagined future to be lived collectively."[36] Indeed, liberals across the ideological spectrum pioneered a broad set of symbols, discourses, rituals, and metaphors that helped construct an idea of a Spanish nation-state in contradistinction to the old regime they were determined to supplant. The role of metaphor in the liberal revolution is of particular interest, given the ubiquity of the "body politic" metaphor, which invited the intervention of politically minded physicians in the conceptual mapping of liberal political culture. It would be inaccurate, however, to think in terms of one, monolithic liberal political culture in Spain; given the aforementioned schisms within Spanish liberalism, it would be more accurate to think in terms of various political subcultures engaged in a series of contentious negotiations over how to define the new polity.[37]

Despite the heterogeneity that would later emerge, one concept that unified early liberalism was the notion of the patria, which was gradually transformed from its former associations with throne and altar into a foundational myth of the Spanish nation.[38] This transformation began with the deaths of Luis Daoíz y Torres and Pedro Velarde y Santillán, two soldiers killed on May 2, 1808, while defending against the French invaders. The popular resistance to the French occupation was by and large carried out under the aegis of the older notion of patria as a territorial entity, rather than the liberal conception of the nation, but on the second anniversary of the deaths of Daoíz and Velarde, the *Dos de Mayo* was proclaimed an annual celebration of "the first martyrs for national liberty."[39] Over the course of the nineteenth century, this new liberal martyrology steadily grew, casting sacrifice in service of the Spanish patria as a symbol not merely of resistance against foreign invaders, but as a blow to the oppressive structures of the old regime and ultimately a down payment toward the creation of a modern, liberal nation-state.

This vision of sacrifice at the altar of an exalted patria was widespread among liberal-minded Spanish physicians, and they often portrayed themselves as long-suffering patriots whose service to the nation was evident in their difficult hours of toil for low pay and scant social recognition, and in their stoicism in the face of danger, whether on the battlefield or at the sickbed. La medicina patria could simply be translated as "medicine of the motherland," or "national medicine," but it could also take on the sense of "patriotic medicine," as in the work of Martínez, wherein he deploys this formulation in a wide-ranging critique of the old regime's scientific backwardness and a celebration of the role of physicians as revolutionary heroes willing to sacrifice themselves for the common good.

Martínez's project was in many respects a historiographic one. His writings on the medical history of Spain, however, were part and parcel of a wider reenvisioning of the past that formed a key element of the liberal revolution. While revolutionary movements inevitably tout their forward-looking visions of progress and emancipation, they also invariably create their own histories, and we can see this in the revisionist history that formed the backdrop for the Spanish liberal revolution. As Richard Herr shows in his seminal work on eighteenth-century Spain, the "birth of the liberal tradition" can be traced to the burgeoning interest in national histories which gained momentum in the Spanish Enlightenment during the reign of Carlos III.[40] It was through these histories that Spanish liberals came to envision themselves as the custodians of a political tradition based upon a medieval constitution that distributed feudal charters and privileges, or *fueros*, among the various classes and regions in Spain, thereby checking the power of the monarchy. For these liberal historians, this tradition represented a golden age of democracy, exemplified by the deliberative council, or *cortes*, which had the distinction of being the first parliamentary body in Western Europe, but ultimately succumbed to royal absolutism under the Habsburg monarchs. This schema in which Habsburg tyranny represented the turning point in Spanish political history, it may be noted, was quite similar to the one outlined by foreign critics of Spain, such as William Prescott. In fact, many liberal intellectuals in Spain, including Ildefonso Martínez, enthusiastically embraced the revisionist "decline and decadence" narrative as a cudgel to wield against the old regime, and in so doing contributed to a discourse that has shaped so much of Spain's conception of itself.[41]

The book is divided into five chapters, the first of which situates Martínez historically in the context of the liberal revolution through his personal writings and the numerous pieces he published in the burgeoning medical press, wherein he held forth on current political affairs and the state of the medical profession. The first chapter also traces the early years in the development of Martínez's career, as he began to make a name for himself through his presentations to a variety of audiences, often assembled at one of the rapidly proliferating medical associations in Madrid.

The second chapter focuses on the assimilation, appropriation, and cooptation of the science of man in nineteenth-century Spain, and in particular the physiology of the passions, which formed a key element of this process. The rise of medicine as a science of man arose within a turbulent mix of competing theories and approaches. In Spain, as elsewhere, battles between these various schools of thought were not fought solely on empirical grounds. Instead, they mobilized deep-seated philosophical, religious, and political commitments, which made such conflicts particularly intense. The physiology of the passions was central to the science of man; indeed, the term "physiology" was often used as a synonym for the science of man itself. A scientific understanding of the passions was seen as crucial to the health of individuals, and to the health of society as a whole, and consequently the discourse on the passions comprised a broad range of topics ranging from the imposition of social discipline to the relationship between the sexes.

Chapter 3 deals with the confrontations between materialism and spiritualism that roiled liberal Spain. The relationship between body and soul was a central theme for the science of man, and a particularly fraught subject in nineteenth-century Europe in general. Debates about the nature of the soul and its relationship to the brain had political ramifications; the naturalizing tendency of Franz Joseph Gall's phrenology, for example, was denounced as a political threat as it subverted the moral accountability necessary to maintain the social order. Ildefonso Martínez was immersed in these debates in true medical-humanist fashion. The early modern treatises that he reissued—Juan Huarte's *Examen de ingenios* and Oliva Sabuco's *Nueva filosofía*—dealt extensively with the brain, and Martínez enlisted them in an attempt to provide an alternative account that would naturalize the soul while bypassing the ethical and political difficulties raised by contemporary mind-body theorizing.

Chapter 4 is an analysis of a central theme in Martínez's *oeuvre:* the physician as martyr. The analysis takes as its point of departure a treatise that Martínez published entitled "Physicians Persecuted by the Spanish Inquisition," in which he appropriates the history of early modern Spanish Inquisition trials involving physicians for the purposes of his own nineteenth-century political project. Martínez's catalog of medical martyrs was an instance of liberal myth-making that functioned as a critique of inquisition, throne, and altar, and as such exemplified the complex and often tendentious uses of the past in attempts to form a new Spanish national identity.

Chapter 5 weaves together a variety of medico-political themes as they played out during the final year of Martínez's life. In 1854, popular uprisings spread throughout Spain, culminating in a revolutionary insurrection in Madrid that toppled the moderate liberal regime in favor of left-wing, progressive rule, while at the same time a virulent outbreak of cholera spread across the Iberian Peninsula. These events produced mutually destabilizing effects: the social disruption brought about by the Revolution of 1854 hampered efforts to contain the epidemic, while the ravages of cholera ensured that the new government would have a difficult time gaining its footing. Against this backdrop, physicians and the medical press confronted a host of contentious issues, ranging from quarantine restrictions and the proper role of government mandates concerning physicians ministering to the sick, to disputes concerning the most advantageous strategies for advancing the fortunes of the medical profession in this new revolutionary reality.

This study of the life of Ildefonso Martínez y Fernández adds to our understanding of liberal Spain in several ways. First, it explores the relationship between early modern and nineteenth-century medico-political literatures in Spain, a relationship that has not been examined in detail before, and argues that Ildefonso Martínez made a significant contribution that has been overlooked. Second, it provides a case study of medicine's role in the creation of novel political cultures in nineteenth-century Spain. Finally, and more broadly, it contributes to our knowledge of a period that has suffered from historiographic neglect, especially in English-language scholarship. The historiography on modern Spain has tended to focus on episodes in which the rest of Europe took an interest in Iberian affairs, such as the Peninsular Wars or the Spanish Civil War, and as a result broad swaths of the nineteenth century have not received the attention they deserve.[42] In particular, the middle decades of the century, when Martínez was professionally active, have yet to be fully explored. Because too little has been written on Ildefonso Martínez in particular, and mid-nineteenth-century Spain in general, I hope this study will serve as a contribution that stimulates future work.

CHAPTER 1

Medical Politics and the Liberal Revolution

Ildefonso Martínez was a significant figure in the medico-political ferment of mid-nineteenth-century Spain. Two means for amplifying medicine's influence in this milieu were professional organizations and medical periodicals, and Martínez stands out in that he founded a number of each. As for professional associations, he founded the Sociedad Médico-Quirúgica de Emulación e Instrucción Recíproca (Medico-Surgical Society for Emulation and Reciprocal Instruction), which subsequently morphed into the Ateneo Médico-Quirúgico Matritense (Medico-Surgical Atheneum of Madrid), and later into the Academia de Esculapio (Academy of Asclepius), and he founded another organization, known as the Instituto Médico de Emulación (Medical Institute for Emulation). As for periodicals, he founded two newspapers that dealt with issues facing the medical profession: *La Verdad* (*The Truth*) and *El Crisol* (*The Crucible*). Via these outlets he undertook a wide range of activities as a public intellectual, serving as gadfly to prominent physicians and politicians, while simultaneously commenting on a broad array of topics ranging from the history of medicine to the latest professional gossip. But in order to fully appreciate Martínez's endeavors, we must have an understanding of the history leading up to his emergence into the public sphere.

A Unique Medico-Political Milieu

The life of Ildefonso Martínez y Fernández was shaped by a distinctive set of circumstances which emerged out of the revolutionary upheavals that reshaped Spanish society during the first half of the nineteenth century, and out of the scientific and medical turmoil that accompanied the demise of the old regime. The catalyst for these developments was the Spanish War of Independence, fought against the French occupation of the peninsula, and the subsequent installation of Joseph Bonaparte on the Spanish throne.

The French invasion of Spain in 1808 had precipitated the abdication of King Carlos IV and opened the way for his son, Fernando VII, to ascend to the throne. Shortly thereafter, however, Fernando fell victim to the machinations of Napoleon, who strong-armed the Spanish monarch into handing over his crown to the emperor's brother, Joseph. But on May 2, a spontaneous uprising in the streets of Madrid against the occupying troops sparked a nationwide revolt, and the French soon found themselves confronted with a hostile populace engaged in guerrilla warfare.[1] The *Dos de Mayo* uprising marked the beginning of the War of Independence, which wreaked havoc as rival armies crisscrossed the peninsula, leaving chaos in their wake, but it also set the stage for unprecedented structural reform and opened the way for the emergence of liberalism in Spain.

The political vacuum left by the departure of Spain's monarchs had been filled by a new governing body, the *Junta Central*, which attempted over the next several years to coordinate military strategy against Napoleon's troops, with mixed success. Early in 1810 the French forces seized the initiative, sweeping through Andalucía and forcing the government to retreat to its last remaining stronghold, the fortified port city of Cádiz. Here the junta was dissolved in favor of a general cortes of the kingdom, which set about drafting a constitution for Spain. Over the next two years, the cortes succeeded in creating one of Europe's most liberal constitutions and undertaking a host of reforms aimed at dismantling the old regime and setting the stage for the consolidation of a new liberal order.

Physicians were well represented among the deputies at the Cortes of Cádiz, and they would go on to assume leadership roles in the decades ahead as subsequent legislative assemblies advanced the liberal revolution. This was not unusual; physicians played similar roles elsewhere in Europe and abroad. Medicine wielded a great deal of cultural authority, combining as it did the twin Enlightenment ideals of scientific rationalism and practical reform, a combination that appealed to the middle-class professionals who made up the vanguard of many liberal nationalist movements.[2] For this audience, medicine qualified as one of the "useful sciences," which Darina Martykánová and Víctor M. Núñez-García have characterized as follows: "These sciences were part of the new way of legitimizing the exercise of power in terms of the rule of reason, and, according to the 'patriotic' elites, provided useful tools to promote the happiness of the nation and the wealth of the country."[3] This characterization captures well the sense of medicina patria as "patriotic medicine," a useful science poised to advance the interests of an emerging liberal coalition.

However, in spite of their conviction that they were fulfilling a patriotic duty, Spanish physicians faced a particularly difficult situation, both politically and medically. The dramatic changes that the new liberal regime sought to impose were controversial among the Spanish masses, and critics never failed to associate them with foreign, French Revolutionary ideals, and thus when the inevitable backlash came, it brought with it a suspicion of foreign influence not only in the realm of politics, but in the realm of medicine and science as well. Combined with this was the moribund state of Spanish medical institutions, which had been in decline even before the chaos unleashed by the French invasion, and were compromised further still by the violent dislocations brought about by revolution and counterrevolution. Medical academies, surgical colleges, laboratories, hospitals, botanical gardens, and anatomical theaters had all been decimated.[4] As a result, during the first third of the nineteenth century, Spanish physicians fought an uphill battle for political and professional reform, a battle characterized by numerous reversals.

The first of these came with the restoration of Fernando VII in 1814. After the French were finally expelled, many Spaniards welcomed Fernando back to the throne in a fit of patriotic fervor as *el rey deseado,* or "the desired one." But Fernando was no friend to liberalism, and as a consequence of his determination to rule as an absolute monarch, many liberal reformers were imprisoned or forced into exile.[5] Among those exiled were a number of prominent physicians whose absence robbed Spain of crucial medical expertise. In many cases the destination of these refugees was France, putting them in closer contact with a Parisian medical establishment that was at the cutting edge of European medical science at the time. This exodus served to create a cadre of émigré physicians schooled in the latest medical teachings, imbued with a cosmopolitan outlook, and eager to return to their home country as medical and political reformers. Their opportunity arrived in 1820 with a revolutionary uprising led by Lieutenant Colonel Rafael del Riego.

One of the most significant legacies of the Peninsular War was a highly politicized military. On the one hand, members of the officer corps had come to embrace a vaunted sense of themselves as the embodiment of the Spanish patria in light of their exploits on the battlefield. On the other hand, the army had become an interest group in its own right, and as such was inclined to support whatever governing faction promised the most generous sinecures and preferments. This combination of idealism and venality created a great deal of political instability throughout the nineteenth century.[6]

The period of the restoration saw various attempts on the part of the military to intervene in civilian affairs. During the War of Independence, many members of the army had been promoted, resulting in a disproportionate number of officers, and any attempt by the monarchy to shrink the bloated ranks of the officer corps was met with ferocious opposition. On several occasions during these years, officers rose up against the government of Fernando VII. Whether out of a sincere affection for the now defunct constitutional order, or out of a sense of professional self-preservation, these attempts to overthrow the monarchy garnered significant support among the military, but in the end they were defeated. The tables were turned, however, in the Revolution of 1820, when Rafael del Riego was able to successfully mobilize the army against the monarchy and force the king to reinstate the Constitution of 1812. Riego's military uprising ushered in the *Trienio Liberal,* during which a hastily assembled new cortes reinstituted the legislation passed by the Cortes of Cádiz and expanded upon it.[7] Physicians were overwhelmingly liberal in political orientation, and many served in the new legislative assembly, like Mateo Seoane Sobral, who emerged as a political leader and strident critic of Fernando VII.

The Revolution of 1820 represented a golden opportunity for the consolidation of liberalism in Spain, and with it the opportunity to improve the fortunes of the medical profession. Operating under a newly established constitutional monarchy, the cortes passed landmark legislation, including a new penal code, a division of the country into uniform provinces on the French model, the abolition of the seigneurial regime, and the abolition of church tithes.[8] The medical establishment took advantage of their political representation in the cortes, drafting a Sanitary Code that was the first of its type in Europe.[9] Outside the cortes, physicians availed themselves of the new freedoms of the Trienio by establishing institutions such as the Medical and Surgical Society of Cádiz, and founding numerous medical journals and publishing houses.

But the gains of the Trienio revealed fissures within the liberal coalition. At the outset, the cortes was dominated by the moderados, well established, elite men of property, many of whom had been active in the revolutionary events of 1812, and these *doceañistas* had gained financially and professionally under the new regime. The exaltados, in contrast, were typically younger, had less of a stake in the status quo, and thus pursued a more radical agenda, which emphasized redistributing property and expanding the franchise. For the moderados, the exaltados were republicans eager to unleash anarchy in the streets; in the eyes of the exaltados, the moderados were, at best, mere opportunists who sought to steer the government toward their own private interests, and at worst, royalist sympathizers. The bitter rivalry between moderados and exaltados, combined with the revolutionary uprisings of Spain's colonies in the Americas, created a chaotic political situation ripe for counterrevolutionary intrigue.

Division among the liberals emboldened the monarchist factions on the right, and by 1823 the country was on the verge of civil war. The actions taken against the Church by the new regime were especially controversial, and the clergy took a leading role in the resistance to the government. Guerrilla bands were formed, sometimes led by actual monks, and in skirmishes government forces managed to kill some of the rebels. Faced with deepening disorder on his southern border, Louis XVIII sent sixty thousand French troops across the frontier to restore Fernando to the throne. Unlike the widespread resistance to the French invasion of 1808, the Spanish populace proved indifferent to the new occupation, and Fernando wasted little time in settling scores, calling for the execution of prominent liberals, which spurred many of them to flee the country. Rafael Riego was captured and later executed on November 9, 1823, in a small plaza in Madrid, after having been paraded through streets lined with jeering crowds.

The modest gains that had been made by the medical classes during the Trienio soon evaporated as the forces of reaction set to work. Because many physicians had been fervent partisans of the liberal cause, the new absolutist regime targeted them as political enemies and came to view the medical profession in general with suspicion. Consequently, many physicians formed part of the wave of liberal refugees seeking asylum abroad. Among them was Mateo Seoane, who fled to London where he learned to speak fluent English, rubbed shoulders with scientific luminaries such as Michael Faraday, and became one of the editors of the scientific and literary journal *The Atheneum*.[10] Those physicians left behind were faced with the grim reality of "the ominous decade," as it came to be known. During this period the assault on the medical sciences was even more dramatic than in previous instances. Medical school faculty suspected of liberal sympathies were purged from Spanish universities, and unqualified political appointees were installed in their places. A draconian censorship was imposed on scientific publications, and in 1824 the government implemented a medical curriculum that designated Latin as the official academic language, mandated the study of the Catholic religion for all students, and recommended a sixteenth-century commentary on the texts of Hippocrates for use in clinical education.[11] Needless to say, these measures did nothing to reverse the marginalization of Spanish medicine from the advances taking place elsewhere in Europe.

Such was the world that awaited Ildefonso Martínez y Fernández when he was born in 1821, in the village of Benia de Onís, in the province of Asturias. Although his family was of modest means, Ildefonso Martínez showed promise at an early age and was sent to Madrid to pursue his education. While in Madrid, Martínez lived temporarily with relatives until he was eventually joined by his father, who opened a tavern in the Plaza Mayor, where Ildefonso worked during his spare time. At fourteen he entered the Royal Academy of San Isidro, where he studied the sciences and humanities, and in 1837, at the age of sixteen, he began his medical training at the Royal College of Medicine and Surgery of San Carlos, and continued his studies until ultimately receiving his doctorate in medicine and surgery in 1844.[12] Upon finishing his studies, Martínez applied for a number of medical posts, with little success, despite his sterling qualifications. Such posts were often granted due to social and political connections rather than medical expertise, and the experience of being denied positions for which he was eminently qualified undoubtedly contributed to Martínez's life-long obsession with corruption and clientage that characterized his political and professional writings. In 1851 Martínez finally managed to secure a position as director of the medicinal baths at Bellús, in the province of Valencia, which due to its seasonal nature allowed Martínez ample time in the offseason to immerse himself in the intellectual and political life of Madrid.

At precisely the time Ildefonso Martínez y Fernández was finishing his schooling and beginning his professional career, Spain was entering what was known as the "moderate decade" (1844–54). The moderate decade, as its name suggests, was dominated by the moderados, who had coalesced into the Moderate Party, and had come to power in yet another *pronunciamiento*, conducted in this instance by General Ramón Narváez. The moderados had been vying for power during the previous years against the *progresistas,* who had taken up the mantle from the exaltados in the years following the demise of the Trienio Liberal and had subsequently emerged as the Progressive Party.[13] After the death of Fernando VII in 1833, a succession crisis had plunged Spain into a bloody, internecine struggle to determine who would ascend to the throne: Fernando's brother, Don Carlos, or his three-year-old daughter, Isabel, under the regency of her mother, María Cristina. The supporters of Don Carlos— the "Carlists," as they were called—championed the traditional privileges of rural Spain against the liberalism of its towns and cities.[14] The conflict was ultimately decided in favor of the liberal defenders of the queen's right to rule as Isabel II, but as was so often the case, out of this liberal victory came renewed factionalism and instability. The Carlist Wars brought to the scene powerful military figures who would dominate Spanish politics in the years to come. One such figure was General Baldomero Espartero, the "sword" of the progresistas, who led a military uprising in 1840 in which he forced María Cristina into exile and took over as regent for Isabel, ruling, in essence, as a caudillo on behalf of the Progressive Party. The ascendancy of the Progressive Party did not last long, however. Faced with the hostility of the moderados to his right and urban unrest on the part of radicalized workers to his left, Espartero was incapable of governing effectively, and in July of 1843 the moderado supporters of María Cristina took their revenge, rallying behind General Ramón Narváez to take over the government and give Espartero a taste of his own medicine, as he, in turn, was forced to flee the country.

The moderate decade witnessed the continuation of the struggle to regenerate Spanish medicine. In the years following the death of Fernando VII, refugees began to trickle back into Spain, including Seoane, for example. But while the political polarization of this period did not approximate that which characterized Fernando's reign, the Moderate Party did not hesitate to censor its ideological opponents, or even exile them if they strayed too far from accepted opinion, either politically or scientifically. Spanish medicine thus remained hamstrung by social divisions and political partisanship and failed to become institutionalized to the same degree as in other European countries.[15]

These twin projects—the regeneration and institutionalization of Spanish medicine—were the work of what José María López Piñero has called the "intermediate generations." The first of these cohorts was made up of scientists and physicians who were born, like Ildefonso Martínez, around the year 1820, and who were responsible for initiating the recovery of Spanish science from its precipitous decline that had resulted from the revolutionary upheavals of the early nineteenth century.[16] It was left to the second intermediate generation, born around 1835, to institutionalize these gains, thereby preparing the way for a "silver age" of scientific production in Spain that took place during the first third of the twentieth century.[17]

The work of these intermediate generations built on earlier attempts to reform medical practice in Spain at the end of the eighteenth century. For example, during the reign of Carlos IV the Royal College of Medicine had been formed in Madrid. The college set professional standards and published an annual list of physicians permitted to practice medicine in the capital.[18] The college disappeared during the War of Independence, and despite renewed efforts to impose similar top-down solutions under Fernando VII, the idea of a centralized "College of Physicians" gave way to a shifting constellation of short-lived medical associations that functioned simultaneously as professional lobbying groups, scientific societies, and political clubs.[19] These associations had a liberal bent, as opposed to the government-sponsored academies and *colegios*, which tended to be more conservative.[20]

The proliferation of medical associations gathered momentum in the late 1830s and early 1840s, at precisely the time Ildefonso Martínez was finishing his medical education, and he became an active promoter of these new professional forums even while still a student. He was a founding member of the Sociedad Médico-Quirúgica de Emulación e Instrucción Recíproca, which underwent several subsequent incarnations, first as the Ateneo Médico-Quirúgico Matritense and later as the Academia de Esculapio. Martínez went on to found the Instituto Médico de Emulación, of which he served as professor and president.

Invitation to a meeting of the Instituto Médico de Emulación.
UCM Biblioteca Histórica Marqués de Valdecilla.

A core function of these associations was the dissemination of medical knowledge via scientific presentations, or *disertaciones,* delivered to the assembled members. The Sociedad Médico-Quirúgica de Emulación e Instrucción Recíproca in its 1839 charter, for example, stated that its members were "unanimously convinced that the sole object of our association is to form a collective body of knowledge out of the individual expertise that we each possess."[21] Toward that end, the society resolved to meet every Saturday to hear a *disertación* presented by one of the members on a topic from the following list:

1. On the general systems of the economy,[22] taking into consideration the ways in which these contribute to the formation of all bodily tissues.
2. On the nervous system in general.
3. On osteogenesis.
4. On the reciprocal influences of solids and liquids on the human body.
5. On the vital principle.
6. On life.

7. On the sympathies.

8. On habit.

9. Causes and phenomena of hunger and thirst.

10. The mechanisms of chemification and chylification.

11. On absorption.

12. On hematosis.

13. On assimilation.

14. On secretions in general.

15. On the secretion of the bile.

16. On pleasure and pain, considered physiologically.

17. On instinct and intelligence.

18. On whether the brain is the material organ of the intelligence.

19. On the conductive action of the nerves in sensation and movement.

20. On affective language.

21. On sleep.

22. On generation.

23. On monstrosities and superfetation.

24. On the temperaments.

25. The physiology of intrauterine life.[23]

Such purely medical topics did not, however, exhaust the themes discussed at the gatherings of the various associations with which Martínez was involved. In keeping with the medico-political nature of these organizations, members held forth on matters related not only to the body, but to the soul as well. In several presentations Martínez dissertated upon the relationship between "the physical and the moral," a topic typical of the "science of man," which had come to exert a powerful influence upon Spanish medicine. On June 21, 1840, at the Ateneo Médico-Quirúgico Matritense, for example, Martínez discussed "the physical, intellectual, and moral education of man."[24] Martínez elaborated further on this theme in a subsequent *disertación* presented at the Ateneo in 1842 entitled "El influjo de lo físico en lo moral y vice-versa" ("The Influence of the Physical on the Moral and Vice-Versa").[25] These investigations into the science of man represent a key aspect of Martínez's medico-political project.

In addition to the role played by medical associations, the rapid profusion of medical periodicals in Spain during this same period had a profound influence on the development of Spanish medicine. As with attempts to professionalize the practice of medicine, the late eighteenth century was a crucial period in the development of periodical literature. Enlightenment-era newspapers in general were hugely popular in Spain, to the extent that the term "journalism" (*periodismo*) gained widespread traction even before the term came into common use in either England or France.[26] But, as was the case with Spanish medical associations, the development of the periodical press was sidetracked by the vicissitudes surrounding the French Revolution and the Spanish War of Independence. It was only in the 1830s and 1840s that periodical literature became permanently ensconced in Spain with the consolidation of the new liberal regime.[27]

In the case of medical periodicals in particular, Spain lagged behind other European countries when it came to their dissemination. As with the periodical press in general, the 1830s and 1840s saw an expansion in medical journals, but in comparison with England, France, or Germany, their numbers were few and they tended to have short lifespans. They were usually either the mouthpiece of a specific medical institution or association, or founded and run by a single individual, or a small group of collaborators.[28]

In September of 1847 Martínez, along with two colleagues, began publishing a medical periodical, *La Verdad: Periódico de Medicina y Ciencias Auxiliares* (*The Truth: Journal of Medicine and the Auxiliary Sciences*). In the paper's inaugural edition, Martínez pointed out the increasingly important role of the periodical press in the dissemination of scientific knowledge: "All the sciences involve immutable, eternal things, such as the divinity from which they emanate; but they also have other aspects which are fleeting, temporary, and subject to the changes and vicissitudes of the times. Who would dispute the right of the periodical press to assist in representing the ebb and flow of ideas, those fluctuations in the opinions of men?"[29] When it came to medicine in particular, the editors lamented "the disgraceful state in which medical professionals find themselves today in Spain, without protection or support," resulting "in no small part from the complete oblivion and indifference with which society views them."[30] They then went on to draw the familiar analogy between the medical profession and the priesthood, an analogy that did not reflect well on the upper echelons of the profession:

Our profession is a priesthood, and we see it as such, and all of our efforts are directed towards instilling this idea in the minds of our young colleagues. But this priesthood resembles a religious calling in more than one respect: peace, charity, consolation of the suffering, support for the invalid, vows of poverty, are practiced by both the parish priest and the village doctor; intrigue, cabals, disdain toward those of a lower rank, no alms for the poor, no allowances made for those unable to pay—this is the conduct of the high-ranking physician, like a canon with a comfortable stipend, living in the lap of luxury.[31]

La Verdad, like so many other medical periodicals during this period, had a brief existence. Not surprisingly, given the tenor of the passage quoted above, the paper made more than its share of enemies among "high-ranking physicians," and it became the subject of several lawsuits filed by parties who had been on the receiving end of *La Verdad*'s scathing critiques.[32] The periodical was faced not only with external animosity, but also with internal tensions, and it lasted barely a year before imploding in a slew of bitter recriminations among its three founding editors.[33]

Martínez, being the ardent polemicist that he was, remained undeterred. At around this same time, he published an article in the *Boletín de Medicina, Cirugía, y Farmacia* (*Bulletin of Medicine, Surgery, and Pharmacy*), in which he took aim, once again, at the perceived shortcomings of Spanish medicine.[34] He lambasted the lax credentialing of physicians in Spain and the corresponding profusion of charlatans and quacks who preyed upon their unwitting patients. Martínez accused these false physicians of "wreaking havoc with their visitations, inflicting grave wrongs, causing deaths, spreading disease and creating hazards" wherever they went.[35] Martínez decried the common practice of bloodletting, which was the favorite treatment of these badly trained pseudo-physicians, who were in his estimation, "the sworn enemies of health."[36] Martínez accused them of being "greedier bloodsuckers than leeches," conducting "bloodletting after bloodletting," and forming part of a "sad, sad profession that torments and kills without restraint."[37]

Martínez took pains to make clear that his criticisms were directed only at those who were abusing the system, not at responsible members of the medical profession, such as "professors of surgery who are honorable gentlemen and only see those patients whom they are authorized and competent to treat." Such figures were not, according to Martínez, "the targets of this diatribe."[38] But of course, this caveat notwithstanding, his critique implicated the profession as a whole insofar as it was responsible for policing its members, and so his critics were quick to pounce. A letter to the editor dated May 11, 1847, and appearing in the *Anales de Cirugía* (*Annals of Surgery*), harshly criticized the *Boletín* for publishing Martínez's "calumnious epithets," demanding that the editors take responsibility for the perceived insult to the medical profession:

> The editors of the *Boletín* know better than I that Martínez does not have sufficient experience as a physician or a surgeon to pass judgment on others. Who does he think he is to criticize so many hardworking professors? It would be utter madness to engage in a polemic with such a contemptible, miserable fellow, with a madman fit to be tied, like this ridiculous Martínez, so I will direct my comments only to the editors of the *Boletín*, who are the ones I hold responsible in this matter; when it comes to a madman such as Martínez, no one should take offense. The best thing to do is tie him up and pity him.[39]

The letter writer went on to mock Martínez's physical appearance, providing the only description that we have of him, although needless to say, one that must be taken with a grain of salt:

> I provide the name of this doctor of medicine and surgery so he will not be confused with anyone else with the same name. The Martínez I am referring to is the son of Pedro Martínez, an innkeeper and bartender at the Tavern of Los Angeles . . . where Doctor Martínez lives. He is of short stature, stoop shouldered, with a broad face; he casts a wide gaze but sees very little; he wears a pince-nez, has a short neck, knock knees, and is a big talker . . . ; let it be understood that I do not mean to mock his physical appearance; each of us is as his parents and God made him.[40]

According to the letter writer, Martínez's article represented a calumny against the entire medical establishment, an underappreciated and poorly paid profession that had sacrificed a great deal for very little reward. Finishing with a sarcastic flourish, the writer suggests that Martínez, residing in a tavern as he did, was perhaps drunk when he wrote the piece: "Do we find here nothing less than a doctor of medical science, breathing the air of a tavern and intoning to the tune of Bacchus his infamous insults?"[41] The letter ends with a warning to the editors of the *Boletín* to be more careful in the future and is signed by one B.S.M., who is identified as an ex-subscriber to the *Boletín*, surgeon of the third class.

The editors of the *Anales de Cirugía* joined in the criticism of Martínez, writing that "in society there are good and bad lawyers, good and bad theologians, good and bad pharmacists, good and bad surgeons, good and bad doctors, whether they have three, five, or seven years of training. Why did the moralizer neglect to mention this? In what medical handbook did he find such insults and epithets?" This bit of editorializing prompted the *Boletín de Medicina, Cirugía, y Farmacia* to join the fray in defense of Martínez. In a subsequent edition of the *Boletín*, the editors wrote: "We deplore that we are forced to answer what was published regarding our paper in the last edition of the *Anales de Cirugía*, but silence could be interpreted as admitting our fault in the matter, and thus we cannot let it pass, despite the fact that in the eyes of any enlightened person, silence would be justified in the face of such a crude and intemperate attack."[42] The editors went on to vouch for Martínez's character, describing him as "upright and well informed," and asserting that "despite his youth, he is deserving of consideration and respect; he has given so many proofs of his education and good judgment that no anonymous insults can possibly make a dent in his reputation."[43]

Once the editors of the *Boletín* had had their say, Martínez took up his own defense, publishing a forceful yet conciliatory manifesto conveying his side of the story. He reiterated that he had clearly directed his comments at a subset of the medical profession, and that he meant no disrespect to physicians who exercised their profession honorably. He then rehearsed his professional bona fides, reminding his readers that he had received outstanding marks as a student, had passed three qualifying exams at the highest level, and had authored several works of literary criticism. In addition, he had been a member of numerous associations, such as the Medical Institute, for which he had served in various administrative capacities, and had been a founding member of the Academy of Asclepius, as well as occupying the chair of "transcendental physiology" therein.[44] The matter was resolved when Martínez and one of the editors of the *Anales*, Salvador Ramos, came to an agreement to retract "all the wording that could be considered injurious either to Sr. Martínez, or the anonymous author—whose name we, as gentlemen, will not reveal." The agreement attested to the fact that Sr. Martínez was "an upright man of exemplary conduct" and "that Don Pedro Martínez, his father, has spared no expense in providing the best and most thorough education for his son," and expressed hope that the accord would bring to an end "this angry polemic" in such a way as "to satisfy both parties and withdraw any words that may have offended the honor of either party."[45]

I highlight these contentious exchanges for two reasons: first, as an example of a public airing of grievances that was typical of the medical press in Spain at the time. As Agustín Albarracín Teulón has noted, "The constant discord among medical professionals during the first two-thirds of the nineteenth century could not help but reveal to the public that those in charge of public and private healthcare constituted a hotbed of discord, disunion, and hostility."[46] Second, because these episodes provide insight into the character of Ildefonso Martínez, whose acerbic style stands out even in the midst of this "hotbed of discord."

Undaunted by the bare-knuckled rhetoric of medical journalism, Martínez founded another periodical, named *El Crisol* (*The Crucible*), in 1855, which blended advocacy for the medical profession with political and literary commentary. As a writer, Martínez adopted a variety of pseudonyms; the masthead of *El Crisol* indicated, for example, that the paper was published "under the direction of Doctor Palomeque." This penchant for pseudonyms seems to have had more to do with a fondness for literary allusions rather than any desire to avoid public scrutiny—Doctor Palomeque was the innkeeper in Cervantes's *Don Quixote*, and Martínez's editorship of *El Crisol* was common knowledge. Articles appeared in *El Crisol* under a number of other pseudonyms, such as *Andanada*, meaning "broadside," or "critique," and *Contreras*, meaning "nonconformist," or "naysayer." It seems Martínez must have had collaborators in this journalistic endeavor because the paper continued publication for a month after his death. Their identities are unknown, however, and this, along with the use of pseudonyms, complicates the attribution of authorship. But many articles published in *El Crisol* are clearly the work of Martínez, as evidenced by their tone and content.

Martínez's signature style, for example, is unmistakable in the inaugural edition of *El Crisol*, which begins with an editorial broadside decrying the sorry state of medical professionals in Spain: "[O]ne breaks out in a cold sweat when viewing the melancholy ruins of the medical edifice, that beautiful bloom which adorns the bouquet of our collective knowledge, which forms a large and important branch of the robust tree of human wisdom. Oh unfortunate nation, that watches indifferently as your most precious temple collapses, that greatest guarantee for curing the bodily afflictions that crush you day in and day out, and offers the most powerful consolation for your downcast spirits!!!"[47]

In a familiar refrain, Martínez blames the situation of the medical classes not on the medical profession itself, but rather on the apathy of a society that did not understand its duty to physicians because it had never had the situation explained properly, which is exactly what *El Crisol* promised to do. What the medical profession needed, according to Martínez, was a periodical that would "faithfully advocate for its positive improvement," one that would highlight the sorry state of Spanish medicine so that "the government and men of means, who are well aware of these ills, will fix their attention on our future."[48]

Liberal Mythmaking

Martínez's membership in an "intermediate generation" of medical professionals was paralleled by his membership in an intermediate generation of liberal political activists. Martínez was at the tail end of a political cohort that had been born too late to take part in the revolutionary events of the early nineteenth century, but too early to form part of a subsequent generation which oversaw the consolidation of constitutional monarchy into a genuine liberal regime in the latter part of the century.[49] While Martínez's generation may not have been present at the creation, it was nevertheless instrumental in the (re)definition and institutionalization of liberalism in Spain that occurred during the 1830s and 1840s.

The relationship of the intermediate political generation to the first generation of liberal reformers was highly contentious; on the one hand, members of this intermediate generation were heirs to the revolutionary achievements of the *doceañistas* and the ideals enshrined in the Constitution of 1812, yet they comprised various factions bitterly divided over the form Spanish liberalism should ultimately take. During this period there emerged an uneasy détente between moderados and progresistas, who joined forces to create a "respectable liberalism" that eschewed revolutionary change in favor of orderly reform, while maintaining differing views on the appropriate speed and scope of that reform. This respectable liberalism was enshrined in the Constitution of 1837, which, in contrast to the Constitution of 1812, created a bicameral legislature that could be dissolved at the whim of the monarch and dramatically limited the franchise to a small group of propertied men. In addition to the Moderate and Progressive parties, a third faction of radical democrats rallied around the Constitution of 1812 and a vision of revolutionary social transformation that repeatedly clashed with the fragile consensus of respectable mainstream liberalism.

Given this wide ideological spectrum, how can we discern where Ildefonso Martínez's political sympathies lay? Fortunately, Martínez was an inveterate commentator on current events, and he read, wrote, and copied numerous treatises on social and political issues; thus, an analysis of his personal papers can provide a sense of his political leanings. Predictably, several of the documents in his personal archive take aim at absolute monarchy. One such document is a copy of an 1833 treatise by renowned *doceañista* Juan Romero Alpuente (1762–1835), written during the succession crisis that set off the first Carlist War. In the treatise, entitled *La sucesión de la corona* (The Succession of the Crown), Romero Alpuente presents a detailed argument for Isabel II's right to rule, and in so doing rehearses many typical liberal political tropes having to do with the definition of legitimate royal authority.

Chief among these was the celebration of elective monarchy practiced in medieval Aragon, which was often contrasted with the royal absolutism that came to characterize Castile.[50] Romero attributes the resurgence of Aragonese sovereignty to the institutions put in place during the reconquest of Spain from the Muslims:

When Spain, having been abandoned by its kings for more than twelve centuries, was forced to take back her territory bit by bit from the Saracens, the first thing that was recovered was her sovereignty. In previous times the kings had been elected by the people, and it was in Aragon that these rights were realized and reinforced, more than in Castile, in the form of a sort of oath required of the kings, which was administered by a tribunal worthy of a free people.

The oath that the Aragonese demanded of their princes was nothing less than the bill of rights of the people and the obligations of the monarchs, and it went as follows: You are no more than any one of us, and we together are greater than you, so do you swear to keep our rights and liberties? "Yes," the king would respond. And then the Aragonese would conclude with this immortal clause: If you guard them you will be our king, but if not, then no.[51]

Here Romero is invoking one of the fundamental legends of Spanish liberalism: that the ancient liberties of the Spanish people—exemplified most fully in the kingdom of Aragon—had been compromised by the imperialism of the Habsburg and Bourbon monarchs, with the complicity of Castile. The tribunal mentioned by Romero was presided over by the *Justicia-Mayor* (Chief Justice) of Aragon, whose job it was to arbitrate disputes between the crown and its subjects. If the king were to bypass this tribunal, the Aragonese would be freed from any obligation to obey him, and could then summon the cortes to elect a new king.[52] Romero goes on to lament the destruction of this check on royal power through the "violence and guile" of the Aragonese monarchs, who gradually converted themselves into demigods in league with the clergy, whom they enriched in exchange for their service. Via this unholy alliance of throne and altar, the people were brutalized into superstitious adulation of their rulers, taking their commands as divine decrees. The clergy, according to Romero, had brainwashed the masses into surrendering their wealth to the church out of fear of eternal damnation and had aided and abetted the kings in "plucking from the crown its most precious jewel, that of elective monarchy, and replacing it with that most dangerous one, hereditary monarchy."[53]

As a fervent supporter of Isabel II, Romero Alpuente rejected the Salic law instituted by Felipe V, the first of the Bourbon monarchs to rule Spain after the War of the Spanish Succession. The Salic law would have prohibited a woman from occupying the Spanish throne, and thus partisans of Isabel favored the *ley de partida*, based on the medieval *Siete Partidas*, which stipulated that women were able to inherit if there were no male heirs, and would thus support Isabel II's claim to the throne. The earlier tradition of succession also had the advantage of predating the ascension of foreign kings to the Spanish throne, and thus coincided with liberal idealizations of the medieval monarchical tradition over and against the foreign Habsburg dynasty. Fernando VII had promulgated the pragmatic sanction in 1830, which drew on his father Carlos IV's unpublished revocation of the Salic law. Romero compares the pragmatic sanction favorably with the ancient law of succession, commenting that it was ratified by the cortes, the voice of the people, and was therefore in keeping with the tradition of the Aragonese Justicia-Mayor with its checks on royal power.[54] After making his case for the rightful succession of Isabel in part one of the treatise, Romero catalogs the dystopian prospects of Spain under the rule of Carlos, the Carlist pretender, noting that he had proven his fanaticism by allowing his daughters to be educated by Jesuits.[55] Don Carlos would rule as an absolute monarch and would follow in the footsteps of his predecessors, who had squandered the royal patrimony with the enormous loss of human capital in the colonization of the New World, in foreign wars in Flanders and elsewhere in Europe, and in "the fanatical and impolitic expulsion of the Moriscos and Jews."[56]

The presence of Romero Alpuente's treatise in Martínez's collected papers suggests that he held some affinity with the author, and in fact Martínez himself penned a forceful denunciation of the conservative royalist party, drawing on arguments put forward by Romero. In a clever rhetorical maneuver, Martínez's essay turns the tables on the royalists, characterizing them as radicals rather than traditionalists. His chief argument against the "royalists or absolutists" is that they falsely present themselves as defenders of "the ancient beliefs of the old society and as representatives of the nation and its historical traditions."[57] Martínez criticizes liberals for taking royalists at their word when they claim to be the guardians of tradition and sets out to show that royalist ideas are not verified by "the sanction of time," and that as a result they are no more venerable than those of other political factions, and that, consequently, royalists are not justified in labeling liberals as "innovators and revolutionaries," when in fact it was the royalists who destroyed "the rights and privileges of the people."[58]

Echoing Romero Alpuente, Martínez rehearses the liberal narrative of elective monarchy, in which "the people elected the head of state from among the most distinguished and virtuous warriors and wise men."[59] Martínez then challenges the royalists: "If the people elected the king and obliged him to obey the laws on penalty of being dethroned, what greater proof of the sovereignty of the nation? Where do we find the divine right?"[60] According to Martínez, claims to divine right on the part of the king are debunked by

Spanish history, a history that "supports the dogma of popular sovereignty resisted so forcefully by the royalists." It is they themselves who are "the revolutionaries and innovators, who in their disdain for that form of government have sought to convert, in the felicitous words of Romero Alpuente, 'the brilliant jewel of elective monarchy into the degraded one of hereditary monarchy.'"[61]

Martínez goes on to invoke another cherished trope of Spanish liberalism: the defeat of the Comuneros at the battle of Villalar. The Comuneros were fighting to defend their traditional privileges against the inroads being made by the new Habsburg dynasty under Charles V. The defeat of the Comuneros and the execution of their leaders were seen as the final blows to the democratic traditions of medieval Spain on the part of a globalizing, centralizing absolute monarchy. Describing the defeat at Villalar, Martínez writes: "the forces of counts and dukes in a monstrous coalition with German troops destroyed those doctrines and their valiant defenders," thus allowing the Austrian Habsburgs to strip Spain of its historic privileges, costing the nation "the loss of all its rights and liberties."[62] The royalists, Martínez warned, should not invoke history in their defense, as their liberal foes will use it against them: "Do not look back past the beginning of this century or we will answer you in all frankness, proving the uselessness of your doctrines and the dangers that they have brought, and will bring, to the nation."[63]

Martínez concludes with a bitter denunciation of the royalist faction, characterizing it as complicit in the illegitimate exercise of monarchical power. The monarch lords over the "lives and possessions of his subjects," according to Martínez, "and even when he is subject to the laws, it is only according to his caprice, given that he reigns and governs, which is to say legislates and executes, without any other power or help when it comes to formulating laws, so he can make or break them and his subjects have no other recourse but to complain respectfully while the monarch remains deaf to their cries."[64] Martínez invokes Louis XIV and his infamous dictum "I am the state," comparing this epitome of absolutism to the machinations of the Spanish Habsburgs: "Here we have absolutism in its genuine form, here we have the institution of Charles I [Charles V] and Felipe II and all the other kings down to our current political regeneration. If they point out that there was a cortes, or the Council of Castile, or the Council of State, we will reply that these were only consultative bodies and subject to the royal veto, that is to say, the royal will, which could laugh in the face of these councils and do whatever it pleased in pursuit of its own interests."[65] Given such royal abuses, there were only two kinds of people that Martínez thought capable of supporting such a political program, the ignorant and the selfish: "the ignorant because of their limited education and the views imposed on them over the course of many centuries," and the selfish, "because they depend on one of those families that has long monopolized the destiny of the nation."[66]

The worst aspect of the royalist faction, according to Martínez, "is that they are of the opinion that no one can or should write, speak, teach, or even think against the established system, and those who do are to be severely punished and made examples of, whether they are peaceful or revolutionary, to the effect that their idea of tolerance can be reduced to the following formula: liberty for my king and church, war to all who write against them."[67] Their only means of maintaining power, Martínez writes, is through "the noose and the penitentiary," because in the end the royalists offer a program that is, "without prestige because it gives no hope, without truth because it fears debate, without justice because it condemns reason, and without rights because one man alone possesses them all."[68]

The Politics of Disaffection

To this point Martínez's political commitments were indistinguishable from the general liberal disdain for absolutism and nostalgia for the elective monarchy of medieval Aragon, but as the moderate decade wore on, his views seem to have radicalized. With the ascendancy of General Narváez, the delicate rapprochement between progresistas and moderados began to unravel in favor of the Moderate Party, which wasted no time in pursuing its advantage. After taking control of the government on May 4, 1844, Narváez secured the election of a pliable new assembly populated overwhelmingly by members of the Moderate Party, which was able to reform the existing political system with the proclamation of a new constitution the following year. The Constitution of 1845 limited civil liberties, disbanded the militias that formed the backbone of progresista power, and officially proclaimed Spain to be a Catholic nation while simultaneously offering financial support to the Church.[69] This period also witnessed an incipient industrialization and fiscal reform that stimulated economic growth and further consolidated power in the hands of the moderados, who were eager to align themselves with the emerging class of wealthy businessmen and captains of industry.

But despite the Moderate Party's control of the assembly, and General Narváez's determination to rule with an iron fist, instability and unrest continued to plague the nation. While Spanish liberalism was riven by conflicts between progresista and moderado factions, these factions themselves were also beset by bitter, internecine strife. The Moderate Party, for example, was plagued with various internal divisions from the *doctrinarios* on the right to the *puritanos* on the left, and these groups failed to agree upon much apart from the need to pursue their own personal interests and advancement in the new political order.[70] Given these simmering tensions, political stability turned out to be a chimera. Narváez attempted to quell divisions in the ranks by clamping down on the press and delaying elections, but he soon fell victim to palace intrigue, having found himself on the wrong side of machinations surrounding the marriage of the queen, and was forced to step down in February of 1846. With Narváez out of the picture, further chaos ensued, and by the spring of 1847 the government was in a state of complete disarray.

Combined with this political disorder was a Europe-wide economic slump which radicalized workers and contributed to the spread of socialist ideas among the younger generation of intellectual elites. It was also during this period that an official Democratic Party began to take shape, attracting disaffected radicals inspired by the exaltados. Against this background Ildefonso Martínez wrote a pair of works that reflect a degree of radicalization absent in the writings we have previously analyzed. In a piece dated May 5, 1847, Martínez proposed a "Project for Universal Emancipation" which sought to mobilize the Spanish masses against the monarchy. The proposed organization would consist of two parts: one public, in the form of a political newspaper, and the other clandestine, in the form of a secret society.

Martínez begins the description of his secret society with a Marxist-inflected class analysis in which he deplores how "kings have co-opted the middle class in their efforts to destroy the liberties of the people, just as they long ago co-opted the aristocracy for the same purpose."[71] In Martínez's estimation, the failure of the common people to mobilize was due to a lack of class solidarity and a false consciousness that gave rise to a "servile adoration" of their oppressors:

Realizing with great regret that the wretchedness, subjugation, and igno-rance of the masses results from a lack of centralization in their work, from a lack of unity in their efforts, and from a lack of education, and above all from their servile adoration of those who are in reality their enemies rather than sincere defenders of the sacrosanct rights and privileges of humanity, we have resolved to make a general call to all those who are passionately committed to following the precious path of the achievements of human-ity, in defense of humanity, in defense of our brethren in doctrine and principle—in short, universal emancipation.[72]

This call was international in scope, relying on "the united efforts of the workers of humanity, of the freemen of all countries, from all nations and all corners of the globe."[73] According to Martínez, the achievement of "universal emancipation" would require an effort that transcended national boundaries: "There exist no nations, no Alps nor Pyrenees, no oceans, no Mediterra-nean—we are all brothers, we are all workers, and we share equally in good fortune and disgrace, in the good and the bad, because we are all working to-ward a common goal: Emancipation, Liberty."[74] Martínez urged his audience to join forces with "the number of citizens who moan and suffer in degra-dation and misery while a few parasites absorb what they produce,"[75] and to form "a society called Universal Emancipation, the sole object of which shall be to increase the sum total of liberty to the greatest extent possible, and to improve in a constant and uniform manner the intellectual, moral, and ma-terial conditions of humanity."[76]

It stands to reason that, having experienced the political repression of the restoration period under Fernando VII, and with it the ever-present possi-bility of imprisonment, exile, or execution, Spanish liberals developed a pen-chant for organizing themselves into secret societies.[77] While such societies existed across the ideological spectrum, they were more prevalent among the factions of the radical left. Martínez's call to "universal emancipation" pro-vides a case in point, as he invokes solidarity with a number of groups on the political far left: "We admit everyone, we preach to everyone, we listen to everyone, we unite everyone under our standard—Carbonari, Masons, Com-munists, Socialists, [and] Comuneros—we summon everyone to the goal of unity in doctrine."[78] All of these groups were part of the radical underground in nineteenth-century Spain.

The Carbonari were originally a secret society of Italian revolutionaries who had been inspired by freemasonry and harbored republican sympathies; their doctrines arrived in Spain via Italian refugees fleeing persecution at home. Freemasonry itself was harshly suppressed in Spain during the restoration but reemerged during the Trienio, when it formed common cause with groups such as the Carbonari and the Society of the Comuneros. The Society of the Comuneros was founded by disaffected exaltados in 1821 and took its name from the sixteenth-century revolt against the efforts of the Habsburg monarch, Charles V, to impose royal absolutism in Spain. Spanish liberals in the nineteenth century saw the Comuneros as kindred spirits in their own struggle against absolute monarchy and made a hero out of Padilla, one of the Comunero leaders who was executed in the aftermath of the revolt. During the 1840s, socialist and communist ideas were beginning to gain a foothold among a new generation of liberal democrats who, like Ildefonso Martínez, were too young to have taken part in the initial clash between liberalism and absolutism in the early years of the century. Socialism and communism, however, were viewed with suspicion by mainstream liberals, and even more so in the wake of the Revolutions of 1848.

The methods of Martínez's proposed organization remain vague, but we can discern in certain passages hints about the possible need for violence in achieving its goals. For example, Martínez writes that the society would avail itself of "war or peace, or elections, in whatever combination necessary to further the goal of universal emancipation."[79] Elsewhere, he seems to countenance the possibility of an armed uprising against the government: "What a grand and powerful achievement, that when taken together, all peoples, the ancients and the moderns, pagans and Christians, share the same universal doctrines, the same pure and sacred principles, and one day they will spring forth with weapons in hand, at the appointed hour, at the same time, directed toward one goal: to overthrow the empire of usurpation and establish equal rights, tolerance, liberty, and the mutually intertwined interests of various peoples as children of a common father."[80]

Given the subversive nature of Martínez's proposal, he took great pains to safeguard the identities of potential participants and to maintain secrecy in the face of widespread use of spies by the government to infiltrate such organizations. For example, he lays out an elaborate branching structure of independent cells comprising three members who would communicate only among themselves while reporting to a central authority, and would remain unknown to the members of other, neighboring cells.

In contrast to the secretive and potentially violent nature of Martínez's political organization, the proposed newspaper would be available to the general public and assumed a tone of high-minded tolerance and avowed a commitment to nonviolent mobilization for social reform. In a second essay, entitled "Democracia, o el porvenir" (Democracy, or the Future), Martínez laid out this idealistic vision of the periodical and described how it would speak to the current political situation: "In the midst of this most crucial of epochs, in these periods of crisis that have been visited upon the Spanish people since the beginning of this century, in these movements and revolutionary convulsions, there has still not been a periodical dedicated to preaching, teaching, and propagating the principles of liberty and [decrying] the excesses of tyranny, without devolving into personal attacks, elevating itself into the sublime field of concepts and sustaining only that which may be sustained through the purity of its principles."[81] Unlike the structure of his secret society, which was based on restricting the flow of information among participants, the newspaper, according to Martínez, would take an ecumenical approach, fostering public debate and seeking out opinions across the political spectrum in hopes of convincing opponents rather than demonizing them. It would "use no weapons apart from reason, and occasional sarcasm, and always with the decorum owed to those who display tolerance for all opinions and respect for all persons" and "debate matters of principle with other periodicals of contrary opinion because there is nothing to fear from doctrines based on other principles, no matter how erroneous and groundless they may seem, because in the crucible of discussion the principles of democracy will stand out just as the sun shines forth amid the dense fog of a winter's day."[82] Martínez assured his readers that "armed only with the weapons of discussion and tolerance you can make an enemy into a friend, and an absolutist into a republican."[83]

The goal of the publication, expressed by Martínez in strikingly religious terms, would be to work toward the triumph of "the interests of the many rather than the few, of rights versus privileges, of integrity over demoralization, of liberty against tyranny, of equality before the law rather than the monopoly of the rich, of enlightenment against ignorance. . . . It is, in the end, the triumph of the evangelical principles of God incarnate against the monopolistic governing principles of political Pharisees, it is ultimately the cause of justice on behalf of the people against the interests and usurpations of crowned heads."[84] The victory of such "evangelical principles" would ultimately amount to "a true communism of ideas, of thought and doctrine," which would "lift a moribund and vilified liberty from the rubble."[85]

The success of this program would require more than mere words, however. Martínez insisted repeatedly on the need for self-discipline, self-abnegation, and nonviolent resistance when confronted with the inevitable pushback on the part of the authorities: "If you suffer persecution for defending your principles, do not abandon them, but rather suffer valiantly in the face of such accusations, and if they are debatable with regard to your principles, do not be so pusillanimous as to turn your back on such an opportunity—have the courage to sustain them in adversity; know that a martyrology is the most solid foundation for the doctrines of the future."[86] Here Martínez introduces a recurrent theme in his writings: martyrdom. A few years later, Martínez would compose his own martyrology of Spanish physicians persecuted by the Inquisition, but here—in contrast with his previous pamphlet, which countenanced the use of violence—he recommends peaceful civil disobedience, and potential martyrdom, as a means of eliciting violence from the authorities in order to discredit the government: "If you are burdened by taxes that have not been ratified by the voters of the nation, refuse them and together form a wall that can only be broken by violence, because violent means bring about the downfall of governments that resort to them."[87]

We have no indication that Martínez's political periodical ever saw the light of day; likewise, there is no evidence that his secret society came to fruition. Of course, absence of evidence is not evidence of absence, especially in the case of a secret society, which by definition seeks to leave as few traces as possible. The proposals do, however, shed light on the evolution of Martínez's political beliefs during the moderate decade. There is no documentation of any formal political affiliation on Martínez's part—with the Democratic Party, for example—but it seems clear from his writings that he had democratic, republican sympathies that situated him well to the left of "respectable liberalism." When it comes to socialism, however, Martínez's views are more difficult to assess. Although he seemed to consider socialism a legitimate option for Spain in his unpublished writings from the 1840s, in later published works he evinced skepticism, referring to socialism as "entirely contrary to morality and science."[88] As to whether he sought to disguise his beliefs in his published work to avoid controversy, or whether his political beliefs were changed by the revolutions of 1848, we can only speculate.

Martínez was undoubtedly a man of the left, but we should be careful to avoid facile categorizations when it comes to the complexity of nineteenth-century Spanish politics. For example, historians have often undertaken a class analysis of the political divisions among Spanish liberals, with the moderados representing financial and landed interests, and the progresistas commerce and the professions, but much of the animus between the various liberal factions was due not to class divisions, but rather to resentment on the part of a younger generation of men who had yet to establish themselves socially and professionally, and consequently found themselves shut off from the "orgy of patronage that had followed the revolution."[89] These men were, more often than not, "office-seekers whose desperate search for preferment and security was to help fuel political change in Spain throughout the nineteenth century."[90] Thus, Martínez's animus toward "high-ranking physicians" and "political Pharisees" may well have stemmed as much from professional resentments as from any consistent class interest. This may also help explain the emphasis on meritocracy among progresistas, an emphasis that formed an important component of progressive political culture.[91]

Similarly, the radical left is often associated with a rejection of Christianity, but while anticlericalism was undoubtedly a fixture among many on the left, there were also powerful religious currents at work in the radical liberalism and republicanism of the 1830s and 1840s. As Genís Barnosell has demonstrated, in the early part of the nineteenth century liberals made a concerted effort to characterize the Constitution of 1812 as the expression of divine will, presenting it as the holy writ of the "God of freedom," a sobriquet that became increasingly common by the time of the Trienio Liberal.[92] This equation of freedom and divinity was thus widespread by the time Martínez was writing his "Project for Universal Emancipation," and it is reflected in his invocation of "the great architect of the universe," and his use of the phrase "God and liberty."[93]

Finally, the relationship between political ideology and medical theorizing has also been prone to overly stark dichotomies, as in López Piñero's assertion that, within the medical profession, the ideological divide between moderates and progressives played out in scientific terms, with moderado physicians tending toward older, vitalist theories, and progresistas championing mechanism, positivism, and experimentalism.[94] As with so much in nineteenth-century Spain, the reality was much more complex, and the career of Ildefonso Martínez y Fernández is a reflection of that complexity.

CHAPTER 2

Spanish Medicine and the Science of Man

The relationship between medicine and politics in nineteenth-century Spain was not limited to the efforts of medical professionals to navigate the new political realities of the emerging liberal regime. While physicians like Ildefonso Martínez y Fernández were politically active during this period, medicine itself had taken on an increasingly political dimension. The late eighteenth century witnessed the rise of an anthropological notion of medicine as an all-encompassing "science of man" that would govern the health not only of individual bodies, but of the body politic as well.[1] This expansive conception of medicine's social role was common throughout Europe. It emerged from the vitalist theorizing of the Montpellier school in France—for example in the Montpellier physician Paul-Joseph Barthez's 1778 treatise *Nouveaux élements de la science de l'homme* (*New Elements of the Science of Man*)—and it remained influential though the first half of the nineteenth century. For example, the German physician Rudolph Virchow, inspired by the revolutions of 1848, outlined an ambitious medico-political program that construed medicine as a social science capable of dramatically improving the human condition.[2] The conception of medicine as a science of man was a pan-European phenomenon, but it took different forms in different national contexts, and the Spanish case has yet to be fully explored.

France was the most salient influence on Spanish medicine in the early decades of the nineteenth century, and thus the reception of the science of man came largely through French sources.[3] As a result, it was inevitably fraught—on the right due to its associations with the French Revolution, and, ironically, on the left because of France's attempts to thwart Spain's liberal revolution.

Ildefonso Martínez y Fernández was forced to negotiate this treacherous ideological terrain as he sought to assimilate the science of man into Spanish medical discourse during the consolidation of the new liberal order.

The Science of Man Crosses the Pyrenees

The science of man was closely related to the science of ideas, or "ideology," associated with figures such as Étienne Bonnot de Condillac, Antoine-Louis-Claude Destutt de Tracy, Jean-Louis-Marc Alibert, and perhaps most famously, Pierre Jean Georges Cabanis. In the second half of the eighteenth century, the tenets of the French "Ideologues" began to filter southward, first into Italy and Portugal, where they were enthusiastically embraced by figures such as Antonio Genovesi and Luis Antonio Verney, whose works were subsequently translated into Spanish.[4] Of all the various Ideologues, Cabanis was especially influential in Spain due to the numerous translations of his books, and the fact that his system was integrated into medical education via a series of reforms undertaken during this period.[5]

For Cabanis and his followers, the "science of man" would unite physiology, psychology, and ethics,[6] as Cabanis declaimed in his 1802 treatise *Rapports du physique et du moral de l'homme* (*On the Relations Between the Physical and Moral Aspects of Man*): "Permit me, therefore, citizens, to address you today on the relations of the physical study of man to the study of the processes of his intellect; on those of the systematic development of his organs with the analogous development of his sentiments and his passions, relations from which it clearly results that physiology, analysis of ideas, and ethics are but the three branches of a single science, which may justly be called THE SCIENCE OF MAN."[7] In elaborating this new science of man, the Ideologues took as their point of departure the sensationalist psychology of Condillac, and were thus committed to the empirical assumptions of Locke, which sought to redefine "metaphysics" as the analysis of mental operations.[8] Where Cabanis departed from the psychology of Condillac was in his insistence that ideas were not merely reflections of external sensations, but rather could arise from within as a result of physiological processes, hence his famous description of thoughts as secretions of the brain.[9] This did not, however, imply a strictly materialist determinism; instead, Cabanis posited a property of "sensitivity" that was an active faculty of matter, and consequently of the human body. Sensitivity represented for Cabanis and his fellow Ideologues a dynamic property that could metamorphose according to differences in age, sex, climate, or exercise.[10] The implication of this position was that physicians could help humans strive toward a healthy equilibrium through appropriate interventions aimed at restoring a balance between individual temperament and environmental factors. The goal of the physician, however, was not limited to merely improving the health of the individual; it was ultimately to improve the species, and society as a whole, and as a result medicine acquired an inescapably political agenda.[11]

In the case of Cabanis, this agenda was bound up with the French Revolution, and as a result it has typically been associated with a materialist, left-wing perspective. For Cabanis the science of man was instrumental to the preservation of the republic, insofar as it served to educate loyal citizens who would be guided by the general will rather than the dictates of the Catholic Church.[12] But as Elizabeth Williams has cautioned, an overemphasis on the personality of Cabanis may result in a distorted view which reduces the medical science of man to a "univocal ideological register."[13] Williams reminds us that the science of man was "a protean, often fragmented discourse" that predated the work of Cabanis in the form of Montpellier vitalism and endured well into the nineteenth century, although scholars have, until relatively recently, neglected this later history: "[T]he neglect of the medical science of man of the early to mid-nineteenth century has stemmed from two interrelated historiographical tendencies: to emphasize the development of forward-looking and progressive rather than traditional or archaic strains of French culture, and to reproduce and valorize ideological antinomies rather than to explore processes of adaptation, accommodation, and co-optation."[14] Williams has detailed these processes of "adaptation, accommodation, and co-optation" in nineteenth-century France, and in Spain similar processes were at work.

The works of Cabanis were banned by the Inquisition in 1819, but inquisitional censorship was notoriously ineffective and they continued to attract a large readership in Spain. They were, however, eventually supplanted by authors keen to adapt the science of man into a form more in keeping with the status quo of "respectable liberalism" and the dictates of the Church. For advocates of the science of man, the passions were a key mediator between the "physical and the moral," and while for Cabanis the passions functioned naturalistically without the need for a special category of mind or soul, later theorists reverted to dualistic notions more compatible with traditional moralism.[15] An influential member of this new cohort of Ideologues was Jean-Louis-Marc Alibert, whose 1825 work *Physiologie des passions ou Nouvelle doctrine des sentiments moraux* (*Physiology of the Passions or a New Doctrine of the Moral Sentiments*) was promptly translated into Spanish and became a touchstone for those seeking to reconcile the science of man with Catholicism.[16] Perhaps an even greater influence on Spanish physicians was Jean-Baptiste Félix Descuret, who pursued a more explicitly religious approach in his *Médecine des passions, ou les passions considérées dans leurs rapports avec les maladies, les lois et la religion* (*The Medicine of the Passions, or the Passions Considered with Regard to Disease, the Law, and Religion*).[17] For Descuret, the passions represented dark, sinful forces to be tamed by man's higher spiritual and intellectual attributes.

The adaptation of the science of man by Spanish writers embraced this vision of the passions, and with it a social agenda in which the masses were associated with unruly urges and dangerous desires. Take, for example, the Catalan physician Pedro Felipe Monlau y Roca, who was the translator of Descuret's *Médecine des passions*. Born in 1808, Monlau had been a left-wing *progresista* in his youth, but had become a conservative *moderado* by the time he published his monumental treatise on public health, *Elementos de higiene pública* (*Elements of Public Hygiene*) in 1847.[18] Monlau's "hygiene" comprised an expansive vision of public health; it shared with the science of man an emphasis on the relation between the physical and the moral, but in this case "the moral" was to be understood exclusively as Christian morality, a morality that the passions threatened to subvert, both on the individual level and the collective: "Nations, like individuals, have their own needs; and nations, like individuals, have, as a consequence, their own passions. A passion is nothing more than a violent, exaggerated need that tyrannizes a man, that dominates him, that perturbs his reason, that sickens his body. And the passions of the masses are likewise nothing more than needs violently satisfied or poorly restrained, that disturb public order, corrupt customs, and are the most terrible obstacle to the good education of nations."[19] Thus, for Monlau, managing the passions is a matter of social hygiene and political necessity; the vices that result from unrestrained passions sicken and corrupt a society and indicate for him that "the precepts of hygiene—which are identical to those of religion and morality—have been violated," and absent a forceful remedy, such corruption will inevitably produce chaos.[20] The "animal passions," described by Monlau inexorably give rise to such vices as gluttony, drunkenness, lust, and sloth. His treatment of sloth (*pereza*) is particularly illuminating, as it reflects the values of an emerging social order in which the accumulation of wealth was seen as a reflection of personal virtue and an avenue to physical well-being: "Without labor, nothing comes to fruition; wealth is nothing other than accumulated labor; and nature made man the sovereign of the universe on the express condition that he labor. Sloth is contrary to the law, to morality, and to public order, and also to the health of the individual. . . . Poverty is the companion of sloth, says the book of Proverbs; and health is the fruit of industriousness."[21] Monlau's vision of medical politics, or "political medicine," as he dubbed it, would require a dramatic reorganization of the state in the form of new legislation, new government bureaucracies, educational reform, and the support of the press in order to enact the changes that "the progress of civilization demands."[22]

A similar perspective can be found in the work of the prominent Galician physician José Varela de Montes, who was a professor of physiology and clinical medicine at the medical school in Santiago, where he was appointed dean in 1850.[23] Like Monlau, Varela presented a vision of the science of man that was steeped in the conservative moderado consensus. Varela offered an analysis of the science of man and its relationship to politics and the passions in an 1834 article, "Fisiología aplicada" (Applied Physiology), published in the *Boletín de Medicina, Cirugía, y Farmacia*. Varela begins with the typical encomium extolling the heroic role of medicine: "In effect, from Hippocrates to Copernicus, Galileo, Locke, Linnaeus, Fourcroy, and Cuvier, there is no aspect of human knowledge that does not owe medicine a great debt of gratitude, as its importance and necessity extend to morality, politics, and the governing of nations."[24] He then suggests that the ultimate goal of all social institutions is the "health and happiness of man," but warns that this must be achieved with the help of a science that "studies his passions and vices, his moral infirmities, which can only be well understood and thereby cured through an understanding of his physical makeup."[25] Continuing along these lines, Varela de Montes describes the science of man as a form of social discipline, beginning with the education of the young: "The principal means of educating of the young should be the correct management of their habits and customs, teaching them to dominate their passions and inclinations, and instructing them in the duties that unite them with their fellow men; and this cannot be achieved without considering the physical nature of man."[26] And he then goes on to outline his political program, with a continued emphasis on discipline and surveillance: "The science of man is believed to have an enormous reach, and this is undoubtedly because it maintains man, and educates him, and governs him—but it must always begin with knowledge of him in order to maintain him, to supervise him, and to govern him."[27]

At this point Varela invokes another central feature of the science of man. In addition to its emphasis on the passions, the science of man stressed the importance of character traits, which could be influenced by factors such as age, sex, nationality, and environment, and could in turn contribute to the health of individuals and societies. In keeping with this focus on character, Varela highlights the importance of environmental factors in determining the habits and customs of a given population. It is only through the painstaking examination of local conditions, and an understanding of the adaptation of the inhabitants to those conditions, that effective governance can proceed: "The common good cannot be adequately pursued apart from a [detailed knowledge of] the localities of the nation, in other words, the spirit and physical disposition of its various peoples."[28] Out of this knowledge comes the possibility of more efficient governing, or as Varela emphasizes, "Let us know men, I repeat, in order to manage them."[29] An added benefit of understanding the inevitable variations between different populations is, according to Varela, that it avoids the danger of assuming a "false equality between the classes."[30] In closing, Varela de Montes proposes that the state should mount a centralized effort to form a cadre of specialized medical functionaries who would study, surveil, and instruct the inhabitants of the various regions of the peninsula in keeping with their particular characteristics: "This is why the principal authorities—political as well as religious—should undertake a detailed study of the inhabitants of the provinces, and also why the central authorities of the nation must have by their side expert representatives assigned to each particular province in order to educate them."[31] The particularism of this interpretation of the science of man is clearly a far cry from the Enlightenment universalism that animated the deputies at the Cortes of Cádiz and the authors of the Constitution of 1812, but it fit well with a respectable liberalism that sought to preserve the existing class structure and avoid social unrest at all costs.

Varela de Montes elaborated at length along these same lines in other works, such as his voluminous *Ensayo de antropología* (*Essay on Anthropology*), and numerous examples of similar treatments by other authors can easily be found.[32] Indeed, recent scholarship has amply documented the ways in which the science of man was adapted in Spain to fit the religious convictions and disciplinary ambitions of moderate liberal reformers.[33] The writings of Ildefonso Martínez y Fernández provide an example of the science of man being not merely adapted, but co-opted to suit the aspirations of an emergent Spanish political culture. In several of his works, Martínez wields the science of man as a weapon with which to attack more conservative medico-political interpretations, and at the same time to defend Spain's national character against foreign criticism.

Patriotic Passions

One of the early conduits of French *idéologie* into Spain was none other than Martínez's mentor, fellow physician, and bibliophile, Bartolomé José Gallardo. Born in 1776, Gallardo was active during the resistance to the French invasion of 1808 and later became the librarian for the Cortes of Cádiz and the author of numerous works notable for their biting satire and anticlericalism. Martínez befriended Gallardo around 1850, whereupon the two men began a brief yet productive literary partnership which culminated in Martinez composing a detailed bibliography of Gallardo's works after his death in 1852.[34]

Gallardo wrote several treatises explicating the doctrines of Cabanis and translated into Spanish an early work by Alibert, the *Discours sur les rapports de la médecine avec les sciences physiques et morales* (*Discourse on the Relationship between Medicine and the Physical and Moral Sciences*).[35] In his prologue to Alibert's treatise, Gallardo rehearses some of the most basic premises of the science of man:

Man must be the target of all the sciences, and especially that of Medicine—of what value are the most exquisite investigations of the properties of bodies if they do not help us better understand humanity, and by extension increase our enjoyments and help us avoid the physical maladies that constantly threaten our bodies as they are continually assaulted by the elements?

From the physical sciences, let us move on to the intellectual and moral sciences, which are nothing without Medicine's assistance. Morality cannot progress apart from Ideology, which in turn cannot progress without the support of physiology. Never has this truth been more evident than in the present day, when it has become the fashion to study the correlation between the physical and the moral.[36]

Indeed, Gallardo's protégé, Ildefonso Martínez, was one of the fashionable theorists who had been studying this correlation; he wrote a pair of treatises on the theme of the relationship between the physical and the moral, which he presented to professional organizations in Madrid. The first of these he read at the Medico-Surgical Atheneum on June 21, 1840. The treatise begins with the requisite paean to the science of man: "Gentlemen, the science that deals with the human realm . . . in its physical, intellectual, and moral relations, is Anthropology, or, the science of man."[37] Martínez goes on to invoke Cabanis and his assertion that physicians, rather than moralists or philosophers, are the ones best suited for this undertaking: "[A]ccording to Cabanis, who is better positioned to understand Man as an intellectual and moral being? Who possesses a better understanding of his needs as a product of his organization, and the means of satisfying them. . . . And where does this knowledge come from? From the actions of our organs and their alterations and modifications by certain agents, that is, from the forces that nature sets in motion, which is exactly what Medicine examines."[38] Martínez then draws on Cabanis once again, citing a passage by Alexander Pope that serves as the epigraph to *Rapports du physique et du moral de l'homme,* and then invoking the Delphic maxim, "know thyself," another favorite of Cabanis:

According to Pope, "the proper study of mankind is man," because only through knowing himself can he come to know his fellow men. From the most remote antiquity this maxim was observed—indeed, we find it inscribed on the frontispiece of the temple at Delphi, with great clarity and concision: "Nosce ipsum," a maxim that should be engraved on the hearts of all mankind as a principle of social harmony, as the source of all human goods, a maxim that should be transmitted from generation to generation, from nation to nation, from person to person, so that in this way it should be as eternal and respected as the eternal existence of the universe.[39]

As a work on the science of man, Martínez's dissertation inevitably dealt with the question of the passions and their proper role in the lives of individuals and societies. But whereas Alibert, Descuret, and their Spanish interpreters, such as Varela de Montes, had recast the passions in traditional terms, as base instincts to be subjugated by man's higher faculties, for Martínez, in accord with earlier Ideologues like Cabanis, the passions were not to be scorned or repressed. Rather, they were to be integrated into a coherent whole: "Nothing is more natural than for a man to have passions and desires; . . . the human passions are the expression of his needs, just like hunger and other sensations, they are necessary . . . for the conservation of the organism."[40] The passions are neither good nor bad, in Martínez's estimation, but rather essential to human flourishing when nurtured wisely and satisfied prudently.

According to Martínez, the process of cultivating the passions takes place on three different levels: the individual, the family, and society as a whole. At the individual level, it is necessary to develop one's talents while at the same time attending to the passions, because "the man who cultivates his intellectual faculties but neglects the regime of the passions is the most unfortunate of all mortals."[41] Within the family, domestic tranquility is to be pursued through the careful assessment of the properties of each family member in order that they may be directed "according to their natural inclinations and shaped by a good education, so that each ends up in a career, art, or trade that best suits their physical, intellectual, and moral faculties."[42]

At the societal level, for Martínez, it is merely a matter of properly deploying the previous two categories—the individual and the family, "because he who is a good father to his family can never fail to be a good citizen, and vice versa." This is the case because societies inevitably reflect the vices and habits of their individual members: "And indeed, it could not be otherwise, because in the end, what is society? It is nothing other than the union of individuals with their temperaments, habits, customs, and idiosyncrasies. And if this is the case, then it is clear that we must begin with the individual in order to reform society; if we wish to reform government it is necessary to begin with ourselves."[43] Martínez goes on to argue that dysfunctional family dynamics can warp a society, and here he quotes Constantin Francois de Volney's assertion that "paternal despotism laid the foundation of despotism in government."[44] It is significant that Martínez invokes another of the Ideologues, and one who exerted a particularly profound influence in Spain. Volney's *The Ruins* had become a classic revolutionary tract. Like the works of Cabanis, Volney's *oeuvre* was banned by the Inquisition, but as in the case of Cabanis, his works continued to be readily available. Volney was a favorite of the radical left in early nineteenth-century Spain, with his scathing analysis of the existing class structure, which he saw as rooted in the power dynamics of the family and as a manifestation of an unjust patriarchy.[45]

The metaphor of the polity as family was common across the political spectrum, and thus Martínez was engaged in a contest of dueling metaphors with monarchists who sought to bolster the claims of Spain's absolute monarchy in support of the old regime by claiming that patriarchy had, in fact, always formed the basis for an orderly civil society. Such an argument was put forth by Lorenzo Hervás y Panduro, for example, who claimed that hierarchy was a crucial element of the social order, and that it had its natural origin in the family with a dominant patriarch at its head. In a passage accompanied by a marginal notation stating that "the essence of hierarchy is found in the society of the family," Hervás y Panduro goes on to elaborate: "The father, in accordance with nature and reason, is superior not only to his children, but also to his consort, for if this were not the case, the family would become a two-headed monstrosity. The mother, who is subject to the father, is certainly superior to the children, who are in turn subordinate to the first born, the immediate successor to the father."[46] In a similar vein, Joaquin Lorenzo Villanueva in his *Catecismo de estado según los principios de la religión* (*Catechism of the State According to the Principles of Religion*) emphasized the role of a hierarchical social order in restraining the unchecked passions that the advocates of absolute monarchy believed would inevitably lead to the downfall of civil society:

> The sons of Adam inherited from our father the love of independence, from which his sin was born. Only through subordination can this tendency be corrected and restrained, thereby preserving us from its damages. This subordination cannot be realized without the existence of a power and authority capable of enforcing it. Thus, no society can endure unless some men are subject to others. Independence and anarchy conspire to bring about

the ruin and dissolution of society. There can be no society where everyone is free to unleash his passions and desires without restraint or fear of punishment.[47]

Thus, for Villanueva it is only religion that has the power to harness the disordered passions wrought by original sin; it is only religion that can, through the quality of charity, provide the necessary cooperation between the members of society, represented here via a venerable metaphor: "The various members of the body politic need each other no less than the members of the natural body; but they lack the true love that impels man to share in the suffering of others, or to provide for his fellow man and give to others part of the fruits of his labor."[48] These metaphors had an intrinsic class element as well. While physicians might differ on the location of the seat of the passions in the human body, when it came to the body politic, the supporters of absolutism agreed that the passions resided among the popular classes. Characteristic of this viewpoint was a work by Manuel Freyre de Castrillón, *Contra el contrato social* (*Against the Social Contract*), which cast popular sovereignty as inescapably subject to the collective passions of the masses. In a passage laced with medical metaphors and similes, Freyre writes: "The masses, having abandoned themselves to their particular interests and passions, distort the meaning of the laws; corrupt the healthiest parts of the administration; replace intelligence with a zeal for power; and like a secret poison that suffocates the first movements of life, they destroy the principles that maintain the function and order of the State."[49]

In Martínez's formulation, in contrast, the passions take on a much different role in the body politic, one more in keeping with an Enlightenment vision that saw the passions not as mere "accidents of the soul," but rather as forces to be productively marshaled.[50] The passions, for Martínez, are not inherently sinful, but rather must be cultivated and directed through a proper education: "To raise a child is to make use of his natural dispositions, his temperament, sensibilities, necessities, and his passions in order to modify and shape them properly, showing him what to love and fear and the means of attaining or avoiding those things."[51] But, alas, the powers that be have shown little interest in this kind of education, according to Martínez. He decries the government's neglect of education, and the nobility's lack of interest as well, but his most bitter invective is reserved for the clergy's monopoly on education, which had inhibited Spain's progress and had been complicit in the imposition of tyranny. Whereas Varela de Montes saw religious authorities as allies in educating the populace, Martínez exhorts them as follows: "And you, minsters of religion, who have for so long been entrusted with the education of the young, cease erecting barriers to human understanding, abandon those of your ilk who work incessantly to introduce despotism and tyranny. . . . Despotic governments fear a good education more than any other weapon that may be raised against them, for, as Licinius once said, education and the sciences are like a deadly cancer to such states."[52]

The antidote to this state of affairs was a tripartite system of education, beginning with a physical education program that would "have the young child exercise his tender organs in order to strengthen them," and this regimen would begin in good sensationalist fashion, with "the external senses, especially those which transmit the most ideas, such as hearing, sight, touch." After this the child would begin his "intellectual education," wherein he would be examined in order to identify his "dominant passion" so that this education could be tailored to fit the individual's particular talents in order to direct him to the appropriate career, rather than following blindly in his father's footsteps. Finally, moral education will direct the passions toward generosity, compassion, and friendship, while eschewing egoism, avarice, vanity, and pride, without a need for religious indoctrination—contrary to the assertions of conservatives such as Villanueva.

The most crucial passion that such an education would stimulate, however, was love of the patria: "But one of the passions that must be cultivated with predilection is that most noble of sentiments, and one of great interest to society: the Love of Country, which is the only passion that I will analyze in particular, not only due to its utility, but also because it will be of interest to my esteemed colleagues."[53] After reviewing older, narrower definitions of patria, Martínez updates the concept in physiological terms. Here he draws on tropes widespread among Spanish liberals, quoting verbatim (but without attribution) the famed *doceañista* Manuel José Quintana, who defined patriotism as a passion produced by the instincts:

Wherever there is Patria, what we find is a passion, an exalted and sublime sentiment produced by instinct, rather than through reflection, that in all cases prefers the interest of the many over that of the individual. It is the eternal source of heroism and prodigious political deeds and the most powerful means of elevating and preserving states. It is a passion to be felt, not defined, to provide inspiration, not to be explained; it is a feeling that expresses more with a single action by a virtuous soul than by all the philosophical expositions, a feeling that demands our admiration, elicits our envy, and leaves in its wake the fervent desire for imitation.[54]

At this point Martínez begins to co-opt the science of man, mobilizing the discourse of the French Ideologues in the service of a patriotic Spanish master narrative. He goes on to invoke familiar examples of patriotic fervor having been brutally extinguished in Spain, such as the heroic deaths of Villalar and Padilla in Castile, and Juan de Lanuza and Pablo Claris in Aragon. Since that time, according to Martínez, there may have been occasional glorious deeds, but none that have risen to the level of authentic patriotism. It was not until May 2, 1808, when the nation, led by Daoíz and Velarde, took up arms against the French invaders, that a new era of patriotism was born—only to be thwarted by the reimposition of absolutism under Fernando VII. But this patriotic passion was not to be extinguished forever; it lay dormant until it was revived by Rafael de Riego during the Liberal Triennium, only to be snuffed out again by the French invasion of 1823. But the force of patriotism can never be destroyed, according to Martínez, because "Patriotism is like a fire, like light or electricity, like any other great force of nature; it is the same for all men."[55]

For Martínez, the science of man and the educational program it entailed were capable of rehabilitating the Spanish patria, allowing Spain to regain its footing among the nations of Europe, and thereby erasing "from the pages of history the derogatory and perfidious maxim of the French, which holds that 'Spain belongs more to Africa than Europe' in the political map of nations, and thus that Spaniards are by nature slaves."[56] In response to this affront to Spanish pride, Martínez mounts a vigorous defense of Spanish culture, noting that while Spain was at the center of the civilized world during the sixteenth century, France was mired in "ignorance and the most idiotic superstitions," and that "before France had a Voltaire and a LaFontaine, Spain had a Calderón and a Lope de Vega, and before there was a Montesquieu, in Spain there was Alfonso the Wise."[57] Martínez then proceeds to rehearse the standard point, made previously by Alpuente, that Spain's democratic institutions predated those of France. But, as the story goes, those democratic institutions, pioneered in Aragon, were corroded over the centuries by power-hungry monarchs and corrupt clergy. He then turns the table on the French, reminding them that in an earlier time they had been a beacon of freedom to oppressed nations, but now have in turn become the oppressors: "You French, who in other times offered oppressed nations the example of liberty, now willfully and recklessly desire that they should help you impose the yoke of slavery."[58] Martínez declares himself "scandalized" by such actions and responds by challenging his audience to embrace the science of man as the key to understanding the "moral principles concerning the nature of man," and thereby facilitate the rebirth of Spain:

> The time is now, my worthy colleagues, you imitators of Aesclepius, to undertake the social regeneration of our Patria, and once the moral principles concerning the nature of man have been instilled you will be able to usher in an era of honor and glory in our wretched Spain! Study in peace, yes, study in peace as the empire of terror has passed away, with its weapons of ignorance that protected the errors of some, the hypocrisy of others, and the superstition of many. The empire of holy liberty has been reborn, which seeks the truth and protects it wherever it is found, without falling into libertinism or irreligion.[59]

After reassuring his listeners that he is not advocating atheism or immorality, Martínez concludes by returning to the familiar theme of martyrdom: "Let us arm ourselves against moral corruption, let us liberate our Patria from the onerous embrace of despotism and tyranny, making of our fragile breasts a rampart, even if it leads to a glorious death in the service of liberating society from the hands of the degenerate and servile. Our names may be erased from the list of the living, but never from the memory of sensible and virtuous men, in whom the sentiment of love of country stirs the heart."[60]

Martínez's appropriation of the science of man for the patriotic project of Spanish national renewal is an example of the "protean" nature of the science of man. Two years later, he reprised many of these themes in a second address to the Atheneum, "Del influjo de lo físico en lo moral y vice-versa" (On the Influence of the Physical on the Moral and Vice-Versa). The address begins in typical fashion by insisting on the relevance of medicine to politics and lamenting the "lack of social analysis on the part of physicians concerning nations and their governments."[61] Central to his analysis is the "influence of the moral on the physical and vice-versa," which according to Martínez is "a subject of great importance and one of the questions that naturally comes into view whenever we contemplate that august sovereign of the universe, man, that most perfect being in the animal hierarchy."[62] And serendipitously for physicians, the recognition of these mutual influences would "bring medicine into the realm of philosophy," and thereby imbue it with a political authority.[63] Ultimately, it falls to physicians to explore these reciprocal influences between the physical and the moral because they are much better suited to the task than "theologians, with their vain suggestions, with their convoluted disputes and incomprehensible mysteries," or "philosophers drunk on their abstract speculations," or "mathematicians occupied with problems and calculations." Through the interventions of medicine, and the patient accumulation of facts, ultimately leading to well-supported theories, physicians will one day be able to "form the ideal image and detailed portrait of man in his physical and moral aspects."[64]

As in his 1840 treatise, education is paramount for Martínez; it is "a second nature that must guide us from the cradle to the grave."[65] Once again, the lack of attention to education by the Spanish state comes under harsh criticism, as it had led to a system in which, "for lack of moral and philosophical education, egoism has trumped the truth and the common good, avarice and demoralization have taken the place of sobriety and virtue."[66] Martínez then charges his medical compatriots with the task of instructing their fellow citizens in the relationship between medicine and "moral and philosophical education," as a means of reforming la medicina patria, invoked here very much in the sense of "patriotic medicine":

> [M]y illustrious colleagues, do not lose heart in your great projects, do not be swayed by the baser passions, but rather shore up the edifice that you yourselves have erected and then build on those solid foundations the fortress of la Medicina Patria, and you will then be truly worthy of her, and worthy of those men in whose veins runs the blood of the Laras, Pelayos, and Zuñigas, and whose souls are still able to elevate themselves toward the heroic deeds of Numancia and Sagunto rather than succumb to chicanery and envy. Yes, colleagues, what I know of you gives me faith in your oaths

and makes clear to me that noble emulation is the flag under which we will fight and never abandon until we have drawn our last breath.[67]

For Martínez, the "solid foundations" upon which la medicina patria was to be built comprised an early modern Spanish medico-political tradition that he sought to revive and update in a nineteenth-century context.

"Spanish Physiology" and Early Modern Medical Politics

Martínez's disquisitions on the science of man were accompanied by writings on the topic of "physiology," which was emerging at the time as an overlapping discourse with the science of man. Cabanis viewed physiology, along with the analysis of ideas and ethics, as an essential element of the science of man.[68] The connotations of the term "physiology" were remarkably fluid during the period; it sometimes functioned as a synonym for the science of man in general, as in the case of Varela de Montes's article on "applied physiology." Indeed, as Juan Rigoli details, beginning in the early nineteenth century, physiology became "a conquering science" which aspired to exclusively describe "the entirety of human experience," and at the same time benefited "from an extraordinary semantic plasticity" that allowed it "to function as a banner of decidedly heterogeneous works without ever completely losing sight of the medical flourishing" that supported it.[69] Given the prestige of this new "conquering science," it makes sense that Ildefonso Martínez, in addition to his writings on the science of man, should take up his pen with regard to physiology. What is particularly significant about Martínez's writings on physiology is not only that they provide another example of an appropriation of the science of man in support of a patriotic Spanish narrative, but also that they intersect with an early modern body of medico-political literature.

Martínez begins his "Treatise on Physiology," with the following typically expansive definition, which emphasizes the role of physiology in regulating the passions in the service of social harmony:

The science that reveals to us man in his natural state goes by the name of Physiology. It is a science that is equally useful to the naturalist, the legislator, the economist, the man of letters, the priest, the citizen, indeed, to all classes of society. To the naturalist it holds forth the promise of perfecting nature itself; to the legislator it reveals the path toward creating laws appropriate to the character and felicity of the society to which he belongs; to the economist it dictates the internal structure of the corporation which he represents; to the man of letters it provides simple descriptions of the most philanthropic customs and entertainments for all classes of society; to the priest, in his role as teacher of the young, it instills in him the most healthy and virtuous sentiments; to the citizen, it indicates the important influence that his social duties exercise upon him, thus differentiating him from idiots and savages; and finally, it [helps] all classes of society to fulfill their duties . . . in order to be useful to the society to which they belong—to stimulate their passions when they are good and restrain them when they are bad, and to satisfy their natural necessities. Having described the utility of physiology, there should be no difficulty in demonstrating the following principle: that the ruin of empires and great nations can be attributed to the ignorance of their peoples with respect to this science, so useful to the rights of society and to liberty, as well as the happiness and well-being of the Patria.[70]

This presentation of physiology feeds into a decidedly liberal worldview in which the rights of the individual are paramount, but are reconcilable with the interests of a harmonious social order:

[T]he moral institutions of society have their origin in the nature of man and his [corporeal] organization; they depend on the life of the individual and the life of the species, and as a result these institutions must first attend to the conservation of the life of the individual and then, secondly, to the life of the species. And since these are the general principles of legislation, we see here the way in which physiology determines the laws; because it is impossible to conceive of how to form a society without these two requirements, which undoubtedly form the essential attributes of the social state. If man does not maintain his own life or that of the species, he cannot conceive life, nor maintain the mutual relationship between different individuals.[71]

For Martínez, unlike respectable liberals such as Varela de Montes and conservative theorists such as Villanueva and Freyre de Castrillón, the social order emerges spontaneously from the nature of man without the need for absolute monarchs or religious authorities to enforce it. Drawing on the sensationalist moral philosophy of the Ideologues, Martínez postulates that "morality itself has its origin in the nature of man due to the law of sensibility, whereby man attains happiness by avoiding pain and seeking pleasure."[72] This hedonic principle does not, however, result in selfishness, but rather in the recognition that it is in the individual's best interest to unite with his fellow citizens to form enduring social bonds because "in unity lies his strength."[73] It is through social cooperation, according to Martínez, that man developed "the ability to observe nature, to navigate the oceans, to cultivate the land and extract metals from the bowels of the earth, to tame the fiercest of animals, and finally, in order to contribute to our happiness by means of legislation."[74] The social solidarity that emerges in a state governed according to the dictates of physiology assures a balance of power and forms a bulwark against tyranny: "Behold how public opinion reaches even to kings upon their thrones, obliging them to contain themselves within the limits of their delegated authority, and all this dependent upon the knowledge of man, or better yet, of his physiology."[75]

To this point, Martínez's gloss on physiology conforms to the standard rhetoric of the science of man, but in another of his unpublished writings he embarks on a historical analysis of what he terms "Spanish physiology." This piece represents another example of creative appropriation, in which he simultaneously celebrates the achievements of Spanish medicine—achievements which in his view have been neglected by the rest of Europe—and critiques the old regime for its censorship of scientific knowledge and persecution of scientists.

Martínez begins with what had become an increasingly common narrative among Spanish progressives, replacing the traditional account of a triumphant Christian reconquest of the Iberian peninsula with a tragic scenario in which a fertile merging of Christian, Islamic, and Jewish cultures was senselessly destroyed.[76] Martínez portrays the Córdoban caliphate as a boon to the sciences, writing that Córdoba under Islamic rule "can be compared to the happiest times in Spain's history."[77] Martínez goes on to praise the library at Córdoba, "the richest in all of Europe," in which were housed "224,000 volumes," and he mentions the "seventy public libraries" in cities such as Murcia, Seville, Toledo, and throughout the rest of the peninsula. Such was the enthusiasm of the Muslims for the sciences, according to Martínez, that one caliph in particular attended scientific lectures with a book under his arm as if he were a mere student himself. With the fall of Granada and the ascension of Fernando and Isabel, the accomplishments of Islamic science went unappreciated, as evidenced by Cardinal Cisneros's order to burn the five thousand manuscripts found in the library of the Alhambra. This regrettable action was driven, in Martínez's estimation, by "fanaticism and a false religious zeal."[78] Likewise, Martínez deplores the expulsion of the Jews, who, having established universities and excelled in the practice of medicine, were unjustly singled out and persecuted for their beliefs. According to Martínez, this sort of religious intolerance was anathema to "philosophers, to humanitarian and philanthropic men, who see those with different religious opinions as nothing other than brothers, as kindred spirits whose divergent beliefs should not cause them to be shunned."[79]

While the ascension of the Catholic Kings may have brought "peace and tranquility" to the realm, it was won at the expense of the sciences, which were inhibited by the looming threat of torture and "the atrocious martyrdom that awaited those unfortunate souls who ran afoul of the clergy."[80] According to Martínez, things went from bad to worse with the arrival of Charles V, the heir to the Habsburg imperial throne, who united Spain and Austria under the aegis of the Holy Roman Empire. The defeat of the Comuneros, the last gasp of democratic resistance to the centralizing tendency of the Habsburg monarchy, together with religious obscurantism, stunted the growth of Spanish physiology: "During this century, many influences conspired to retard the progress of science, and even more so that of physiology, the branch of medicine which requires the greatest freedom for its discussions, and which found itself smothered by inquisitorial despotism. One had to find a powerful patron at court—a saint, or a cleric, or a bishop, or perhaps a familiar of the Inquisition—in order to publish one's doctrines, covering them always with a veil of religious mysticism and supporting them with references to sacred texts."[81] Martínez concludes his historical reflection with a lament for what might have been, had the Church not oppressed Spanish authors in this way. He pleads for understanding from the rest of Europe when judging the merits of Spanish thinkers, who, in his estimation, should be admired for the work they did in the face of threats of torture and execution.

After acknowledging these considerable barriers to scientific advancement, Martínez lays claim to a unique medico-political tradition in early modern Spain that related insights from the practice of medicine and the study of human anatomy to ethics, art, and political theory. According to Martínez, Spanish philosophers during this era were well versed in "the application of anatomy to moral theology, sculpture, and politics."[82] Indeed, from the late sixteenth century onward, medicine came to play an increasingly important part in Spanish culture, and as Jon Arrizabalaga has argued, "a prescriptive role in the politics of the Spanish crown."[83] During this time there developed a genre of medico-political literature that sought not only to delineate proper conduct for individual physicians but also to elaborate upon the proper relations between medical science and political philosophy. All of these works grew not only out of a preoccupation with the reform of medical education and practice, but also out of a growing interest in the role of medicine in governance and social policy. In addition, these works were vibrant repositories for organicist metaphors pertaining to the body politic, and thus contributed to the formation of the political culture of early modern Spain.

Martínez mentions in particular the physician Jerónimo Merola, whose *República sacada del cuerpo de hombre* (*Republic Based on the Human Body*) was a classic exemplar of this genre of medico-political literature. Merola published his treatise in 1587 and went on to produce two more editions, one in 1595 and another in 1611. Merola was around the age of fifty when he wrote the book; he had left his native Barcelona to study medicine at Montpellier under the medical humanist Guillaume Rondelet, who was a champion of Vesalius's experimental anatomy. Upon finishing his studies at Montpellier, Merola returned to his native city to take up a post as professor of medicine at the University of Barcelona.[84]

Merola's text employs an analogy between the human body and a proper political order, drawing heavily on earlier thinkers, such as Plato and John of Salisbury, but at the same time bringing a Renaissance perspective to the classic body politic metaphor.[85] Like Cabanis, Merola invokes in his prologue the Delphic maxim "know thyself," implying that by turning our gaze inward we find the natural structure of society. Merola's ideal political order is a hierarchical one in which each member plays a specific role, just as the components of the human body must act in perfect concert to preserve health:

In a kingdom the King governs, and he has below him subordinates who obey according to reason and the law: and towards them he exercises justice, always gently and with great mercy, and he has Princes and grandees through whom he governs, relying on them in times of peace and in times of war. . . . Likewise the human body is justly ruled and governed by nature, which like a King, ensures that no part of the body causes injury nor takes what does not belong to it; rather, [nature] infuses it with heat and spirits, and inspires it in such a way that they obey and acknowledge her in both times of peace and of war (which is to say, in times of health and in times of illness).[86]

Merola breaks his analogy down into the traditional tripartite division between head, heart, and liver, which correspond to the "architects" of the republic: theologians, physicians, and jurists respectively. The brain symbolizes the role of the theologians in directing the body politic toward virtue, but this is only possible due to the blood supplied by the heart, which carries the animal spirits necessary for the brain to function. The duty of the physician in Merola's metaphorical schema is to nurture the republic by ministering to its citizens, keeping them healthy and productive. Jurists, in turn, correspond to the liver because this is the organ—in Merola's version of Galenic physiology—that breaks down food into blood and then distributes blood to the various organs of the body, including the heart, just as jurists occupy themselves with distributing the basic goods of society among its members.

At first glance, Merola's republic is organized hierarchically; such hierarchical schemas were common in the late sixteenth century, given the confluence during the period of Neo-Platonism, Roman law, and Counter-Reformation statecraft, but as Augustine Redondo observes, Merola's body politic metaphor deviates from the orthodox model insofar as it privileges men of letters over a hereditary aristocracy. Aristocrats are reduced to the status of parasites that leach off the body politic.[87] So Merola is actively, it seems, shifting the emphasis of the body politic metaphor from inherited hierarchy to meritocracy. In Merola's estimation, the obsession with "honor" among the nobility is antithetical to a truly Christian society in which honor is given to those who subordinate their individual will to the common good. Merola lauds those who, although they may start from a lower estate, through effort and education rise above "princes and men of advantageous fortune." Conversely, for Merola, kings, dukes, and doctors of philosophy should be counted among the plebeians if their opinions and behavior merit it.[88] Ultimately, men must be measured by "what is of the best and of greatest value in them, which are the things of the spirit and the understanding, and not what they have received from fickle fortune."[89] According to Merola, physicians take pride of place in the republic, over and above jurists, who merely deal with "fortune," that is, the distribution of worldly goods necessary to keep the plebeians satisfied; physicians, in contrast, are concerned with the health of the body politic, playing a vital function, like the heart, maintaining balance and providing nourishment to all its members.

This celebration of physicians was in keeping with another type of medico-political work dedicated to extolling the virtues of the medical classes: the "mirror of the physician." A prominent example of this genre is Enríque Jorge Enriquez's *Retrato del perfecto médico* (*Portrait of the Perfect Physician*), published in 1595. The book is structured as a dialogue between two "architects," as in Merola's schema: the author, a physician, and a theologian who serves as his interlocutor. Also in keeping with Merola's approach, Enríquez takes an explicitly Platonic tack, seeking to measure contemporary physicians according to an ideal that specified a male, Catholic, university-trained exemplar.[90] Those who departed from this ideal, such as women healers, came under fierce criticism. Enríquez also decries the corruption of authorities who fill offices not with the most learned and qualified, but rather with "illiterates" and "idiots."[91]

It stands to reason that such exemplars of early modern medico-political literature held an attraction for Ildefonso Martínez; both Enríquez and Merola lived through particularly turbulent political epochs, as did Martínez, and they both portrayed physicians as necessary for diagnosing and curing the ills of the body politic, as did the science of man during the eighteenth and nineteenth centuries. They both endorsed a meritocratic social order in which physicians played a crucial role and advocated for the professionalization of medicine and the improved treatment of physicians as a class—themes that resonated into the nineteenth century. But the two most important early modern thinkers for Martínez's interventions into the medico-political debates of the nineteenth-century were Juan Huarte de San Juan and Oliva Sabuco de Nantes Barrera.

Huarte's celebrated book, the *Examen de ingenios* (*The Examination of Men's Wits*), first published in 1575, was a landmark in the history of psychology, representing the first attempt to account for psychological differences, and differences in aptitudes, in purely physiological terms. The *Examen* was translated into many languages and circulated throughout Europe, but the book's perceived determinism and naturalism were hard to align with Catholic doctrine on free will and the immortality of the soul, and consequently it was condemned by the Spanish Inquisition and was reissued in a revised edition in 1594.[92] Oliva Sabuco de Nantes Barrera was the author of *Nueva filosofía de la naturaleza del hombre* (*New Philosophy of Human Nature*), published in 1587, the same year as Merola's *República sacada del cuerpo de hombre*. Like Huarte, Oliva Sabuco addressed the mind-body problem in a radical new fashion for her time, and as in the case of Huarte, Sabuco's *Nueva filosofía* attracted the attention of the Holy Office and had to be reissued in a slightly expurgated version. In an attempt to right what he perceived to be a historical injustice, Martínez produced in 1845 a new Spanish edition of Huarte's *Examen,* restored for the first time to its original, unexpurgated form, and two years later he came out with a new edition of Sabuco's *Nueva filosofía.*[93]

Huarte and Sabuco were both innovative natural philosophers who proposed groundbreaking physiological accounts of psychological phenomena, and neither was shy when it came to proclaiming the political implications of their work; both authors prefaced their treatises with dedicatory epistles to King Felipe II himself, arguing that their prescriptions for the health of individuals would benefit society as a whole.[94] Huarte's differential psychology, with its promise of identifying specific aptitudes among the king's subjects, could be a guide to the reform of education by matching students with the courses of study and career choices most suitable for them, which would make for a more efficient use of human resources and thereby fortify the state.[95] Sabuco, in turn, offered an account of how the passions generated by the brain influence physical and mental health, and how, armed with this knowledge, rulers could gain a better understanding of "the nature and the attributes of men," so as to "know better how to rule them and govern their world."[96]

In many respects, Huarte and Sabuco represented for Martínez a matched pair of resources to link the genius of early modern Spanish medico-political theorizing with contemporary debates on the science of man.[97] Unlike Huarte, however, Sabuco was a woman, and gender constituted a through line within early modern and late modern medico-political discourses that culminated in the professionalization of medicine in the nineteenth century, when the science of man was instrumental in medicine becoming quite literally a masculine science.

The Science of Man and Men of Science

The science of man took great interest in the influence of physiological characteristics on personality traits, and a favorite target of this interest was gender. Cabanis dedicated the Fifth Memoir of the *Rapports* to "The Influences of the Sexes on the Character of the Ideas and of the Moral Affections," and in this memoir he presents his version of female physiology in an attempt to naturalize the social roles of the sexes, attributing to women an emotional pliability that was determined by the literal pliability of their tissues:

> Through a strict necessity related to the role assigned to her by nature, the woman finds herself subject to many accidents and inconveniences. Her life is almost always a sequence of alternates of well-being and of suffering, in which too often suffering dominates. Thus her fibers have to be pliant enough to make her capable of these continual frictions. Their contractility must be less strong, though acute and prompt, in order to be able to bring them back to their average state immediately. It is also, and even more, necessary that the general sensibility have the same character of promptness and acuteness that makes it capable of resuming its natural tone easily, after having ceded without resistance to all impressions, after having let itself be pushed, as it were, to all extremes, either of excess or of privation. To add to the sweet seduction of the sex and of beauty, does nature not seem even to have provided the woman be put in a customary state of relative weakness? The main grace of man is his vigor. The power of woman is hidden in more delicate means; one does not want her to be so strong.[98]

Given their inherent debility, it is axiomatic for Cabanis that women should not participate in the public sphere:

Because of her weakness, the woman, wherever the tyranny and the prejudices of men have not forced her to violate her nature, has had to remain inside the house or the hut. Particular inconveniences and the care of the children retained her there, or unceasingly brought her back. She had to make of this stay a habit. Incapable of supporting the fatigues, of affronting the dangers, of resisting the tumultuous shock of great assemblies of men, she left to them the hard work and the dangers they had chosen by preference. She did not mingle in discussions of public affairs, at which not only must there always preside a severe and strong reason, but where also the accent of the character and energy add singularly to the power of reason. She reserved herself to the interior cares of the family and that gentle domestic empire by which alone she becomes at once respectable and touching.[99]

Ildefonso Martínez took a similarly sexist line with regard to differences between men and women. In his treatise "On the Influence of the Physical on the Moral and Vice-Versa," he characterizes women as the weaker sex, both physically and intellectually, asserting that "the world of men is one of abstraction and speculation, one that is not accessible to women."[100] Women are, according to Martínez, "timid, cunning, jealous, fickle, compassionate, charitable, and superstitious."[101] This insistence on a stark polarity between the sexes was another instance in which Martínez could draw parallels between early modern medico-political literature and the science of man. Juan Huarte in his *Examen* provided a biologically deterministic explanation of the differences in aptitudes between the sexes that came to conclusions similar to those of Cabanis, even though those conclusions derived from very different physiological assumptions.

Huarte's theory of the *ingenios*, or "wits," took as its point of departure the reigning Aristotelian Galenism of the day and applied it to the brain in order to explain variances in cognitive ability. Huarte drew on the theory of temperament, that is to say the relationship between hot, cold, dry, and moist and their accompanying elements: air, fire, earth, and water, as they combined to produce the four humors: blood, phlegm, yellow bile, and black bile.[102] The balance of these humors in any given person affected the composition of the brain, which then determined the limits of that individual's intellectual development. Women, in Huarte's schema, were cold and moist in temperament, and were consequently less intelligent: "Females cannot attain great intelligence due to the coldness and moisture of their sex; they are only able to give the appearance of ability when treating superficial, simple subjects and using common, clichéd language; when it comes to academic work, they are able to learn a little Latin, but merely because this only requires memory. We should not blame them for these failings, however, because they are due to the coldness and moisture of women's nature, which as we have seen, work against intelligence and ability."[103] In his notes to the *Examen,* Martínez echoes Huarte's misogyny, writing that "women are not suited for the vast majority of the sciences, and this is a result not only of their moral and political education, but also of their physical makeup, which is very different from that of men."[104] Elsewhere, however, he warns that such characterizations "must be taken in a general sense, not in an absolute sense," because "there are important exceptions."[105] Martínez then goes on to cite numerous women who have excelled in the arts and sciences, and among these he lists Oliva Sabuco.

Oliva Sabuco Barrera de Nantes was born in 1562, the daughter of Miguel Sabuco, who is thought to have been an apothecary in the town of Alcaraz, located in the archdiocese of Toledo.[106] When, at the age of twenty-five, Oliva Sabuco produced her *Nueva filosofía,* she was immediately lauded as a leading light among Spanish natural philosophers. Ildefonso Martínez announced his forthcoming version of Sabuco's *Nueva filosofía* in September of 1847, in the inaugural edition of his newspaper, *La Verdad,* writing that the publication of Sabuco's treatise was part of his larger project of reissuing classic works from the history of Spanish science. Although the celebrated historians of medicine Antonio Hernández Morejón and Anastasio Chinchilla y Piqueras had recently published voluminous biblio-biographical treatments of the history of Spanish medicine, Martínez felt that their works, which consisted of brief biographies of Spanish physicians in chronological order, were not sufficient to restore the prestige of Spanish medicine. Instead, Martínez was committed to publishing an eclectic selection of key contributions to the history of Spanish medicine, and chief among these "monuments of literary glory" would be the *Nueva filosofía de la naturaleza del hombre,* authored by "an honorable lady of our literary history."[107]

Despite this praise directed at Sabuco, when the new edition of the *Nueva filosofía* came out later that year, Martínez expressed skepticism in his introduction as to whether a woman could have actually authored such an extraordinary piece of scholarship: "[S]uch is the eloquence of the author, in both Spanish and Latin, it is no wonder that the more one studies this production, the more one is convinced that it was a man rather than a woman who wrote this most beautiful work."[108] He goes on to quote Anastasio Chinchilla, who expressed similar doubts, writing that "it is difficult to believe that a woman could have been so expert in the sciences," and asking how a woman of such erudition could have gone unremarked upon at the time.[109]

Despite such periodic skepticism, there was no serious challenge to Oliva Sabuco's authorship of the *New Philosophy* until 1903, when documents were discovered purporting to show that Oliva's father, Miguel Sabuco, had actually written the work. Despite the ambiguity of the evidence, many library catalogues transferred authorship of the work to Miguel Sabuco, but historians continue to debate the issue. Mary Ellen Waithe and Maria Colomer Vintró, for example, claim to have definitively proved that Oliva Sabuco was wrongly stripped of her authorship, while Gianna Pomata insists that the facts remain in dispute.[110]

Ildefonso Martínez, of course, was not privy to this later controversy concerning the authorship of the *Nueva filosofía,* and he concludes his introduction by giving the last word to Martín Martínez, the editor of an early eighteenth-century version of the work, who professed his belief in Oliva's authorship, citing the huge risk of falsifying the authorship of such a prominent work as the *Nueva filosofía,* especially given that it was dedicated to Felipe II, king of Spain: "There are those who say that this work was not written by a woman, but I am not persuaded of this because the sovereign to whom the work was dedicated was so grave and circumspect that when it comes to such serious and important material, no one would have dared to deceive him."[111] Despite his initial skepticism, Ildefonso Martínez seems to have concurred with Martín Martínez and refers throughout his writings to "Doña Oliva" as the author of the *Nueva filosofía* and as a "heroine" of Spanish science.

The strategy initially proposed by Martínez with regard to the publication of Sabuco's work was to reissue only the first chapter of the *Nueva filosofía,* on the "philosophy of the passions,"[112] entitled "Conocimiento de sí mismo" (Knowledge of Oneself), thereby producing a "philosophical edition rather than a simple reissue."[113] In the end, Martínez also included another chapter of medico-political significance, "Things That Will Improve This World and

Its Nations," but the main emphasis in his annotations to the work remained on Sabuco's treatment of the passions, which Martínez compared favorably to those of celebrated expositors of the science of man, such as Alibert.

Ironically, while Martínez was championing a woman's medico-political treatise on the passions, the passions were becoming increasingly central to the emergence of scientific masculinity in the nineteenth century, a development that contributed to the marginalization of women from the medical profession. As Darina Martykánová and Víctor Núñez-García have shown, Spanish physicians were increasingly committed to a form of "Romantic masculinity" that privileged not merely rationality, but also the passions, which were to be employed in such a way as to benefit the patria, as well as humanity in general.[114] The professionalization of medicine in Spain was a process through which physicians emerged on the one hand as reasonable "men of science," and on the other, as passionate "lovers of humanity" who were willing to sacrifice themselves for the public good.

Such a conception of Romantic masculinity fits remarkably well with Martínez's treatment of the passions and his evocation of a "patriotic medicine." This conception entailed not only service to the medical profession, but public service as well, as evidenced by the exalted patriotism expressed by so many physicians in the medical press, and the countless tracts extolling the value of medicine to the state, which often translated into calls for physicians to seek public office. We find such an exhortation in the pages of *El Siglo Médico* in an article that applauded efforts aimed at installing physicians in political office at the provincial level as a means of destroying "the mistaken idea that physicians serve only to cure the sick."[115] In keeping with the medical profession's increasingly expansive self-image, such efforts were characterized as directed toward "neither personal aggrandizement, nor a ridiculous class privilege, but rather above all the general welfare." Through political participation, physicians would "achieve the social position that is their right, and that is so necessary in order for them to labor for the happiness of humanity."[116]

Martínez's repeated calls for self-sacrifice in the service of medicine are another example of this form of Romantic masculinity. Martínez characterizes medicine as the "the most difficult, the most noble, the most sublime of the sciences, but also the most miserable, in which rose petals alternate with thorns, joys with sorrows, pleasures with sadness," and then goes on to warn aspiring physicians that the practice of medicine requires a commitment to selfless public service that will inevitably go unappreciated, and that "the only reward for your efforts will be the ingratitude of your fellow men, continual agitation, a middling social status, the disillusionments caused by your impotence, and the melancholy satisfaction of having done your duty."[117] A medical vocation, for Martínez, demands pure motives and a willingness to undergo extreme self-abnegation to the point of martyrdom:[118]

> Happiness unto you if a true calling and talent guide you toward this great enterprise! Misery if self-interest and ambition are your motives! Yes, my friends; if you are firmly disposed to suffer greatly in order to know little, to face danger only to experience disappointment, to live as martyrs in order to die virtuously, to spend your patrimony without reimbursement, then enter into the temple; but if you are weak, if you are unable to resist temptation, if you do not know the virtue of heroism and the duty of sacrifice, then retreat, do not profane the temple of Asclepius.[119]

Such dramatic warnings about the rigors of medical practice certainly conjured up Romantic images of sacrificial heroism among physicians, but they also served to exclude women from the practice of medicine. Women were increasingly being relegated to the domestic sphere in the emerging liberal order, where they were simultaneously marginalized and idealized as *ángeles del hogar* (angels of the home).[120] Descriptions of the life of a physician inevitably emphasized not only the arduous training and low pay, but also the need to travel over long distances day and night in order to treat patients in their homes, which further served to masculinize the profession, as women were discouraged by the standards of bourgeois respectability from traveling independently or entering a stranger's house unaccompanied.[121] It is also telling that, as the role of women was being circumscribed within the domestic sphere, the role of the physician was expanding to include political activism in the public sphere.

All of these trends were in keeping with a general marginalization of women from medicine that began during the early modern era of Oliva Sabuco and culminated in the nineteenth century.[122] In Spain, for example, the profession was transformed during the nineteenth century into an exclusively male province, the admission to which was controlled by the requirement of a university degree and a regimen of increasingly strict professional regulations and certifications that effectively excluded women healers.[123] In addition, the conceptualization of medicine as an exclusively masculine pursuit corresponded with the emergence of male-only spaces dedicated to disseminating medical knowledge, such as Martínez's Sociedad Médico-Quirúgica de Emulación, modeled after the Société Médicale d'Emulation, founded by Jean-Louis Alibert in 1796. The emphasis here on emulation is significant, according to Martykánová and Núñez García, because it showed that Romantic masculinity was not individualistic, but rather a collective pursuit: "Emulation was the key dynamic: men were to emulate those who had distinguished themselves through their own merit—they were expected to overcome every manner of obstacle, and as a reward for their efforts, they would in turn be emulated by others."[124] This mutually reinforcing cycle of social recognition is evoked in Martínez's previously quoted exhortation to his colleagues in which he declares that "emulation is the flag under which we will fight and never abandon until we have drawn our last breath."[125]

CHAPTER 3

On the Matter of Mind

As described in the last chapter, there existed an early modern corpus of medico-political literature in Spain geared toward integrating medicine with social and political reform, and this corpus exerted a powerful influence on Ildefonso Martínez's engagement with the science of man. A central theme of this literature was a preference for naturalistic explanations of mental phenomena and an attendant interest in analyzing the structures and functions of the brain. This theme was especially salient in the works of Oliva Sabuco and Juan Huarte that Martínez reissued. When Martínez produced his editions of *La nueva filosofía* and *El examen de ingenios,* he was not acting out of purely antiquarian motives, but rather seeking to address contemporary concerns and contribute to a specific intellectual agenda.

The period of revolutions spanning the late eighteenth and early nineteenth centuries was not merely about politics; it was also about revolutionary new ways of conceiving the mind-brain. Indeed, these dual revolutions were intimately connected: notions concerning the mind's materiality, or lack thereof, were bound up in political disputes over the nature of the soul, the existence of free will, moral accountability, and the capacity for self-government. The materialist theories of Ideologues such as Pierre Jean Georges Cabanis emerged out of the dismantling of the old regime in France, and were consequently associated with revolutionary politics. Elsewhere in Europe, similarly thoroughgoing revisions of the nature of mind were undertaken by figures such as Franz Joseph Gall in Germany and Erasmus Darwin in England. Such thinkers exemplified the interconnections between politics and psychology, as their doctrines were likewise associated in the public imagination with a "radical science" that threatened to undermine the verities of late-eighteenth- and early nineteenth-century polite society.

Spain was by no means immune to these controversies. The liberal revolution contained within it contrasting ideological tendencies, and these played out among Spanish physicians in their disputes over the implications of materialism and spiritualism. As was the case elsewhere in Europe, these disputes often broke down along partisan lines, with materialists tending leftward and spiritualists rightward, but we should avoid oversimplifying this dichotomy. The example of Ildefonso Martínez y Fernández provides a case in point. Despite his left-leaning political stance, Martínez took a nuanced position in these debates, a position located in the middle ground between what he considered to be the excesses of both materialism and spiritualism.

The Liberal Soul

In Spain during the early decades of the nineteenth century, debates about the nature of the soul became particularly intense as numerous tracts on the mind-body relationship were translated into Spanish, including works by Darwin, Gall, and Cabanis. The psychologies put forward by these three writers have been construed by Alan Richardson as bearing a family resemblance. These thinkers, while not constituting a formal school of any kind, did, in Richardson's estimation, make up a "constellation of roughly affiliated theoretical positions" that shared a number of assumptions: "All of them agree in locating the mind in the brain, the 'cerebral organ' or organ of thought. They all emphasize that the mind is an active processor, rather than a passive register of experience, holding this in common with German idealist philosophy and with Scottish 'common sense' psychology but uniquely seeking to elucidate the active mind in neurological terms. . . . They all stress the complexity of the brain, often envisioning it as a collection of organs."[1] The radical implications of this strain of thought were anathema to the mid-century moderado consensus, a consensus committed to the teachings of the Catholic Church and the bourgeois status quo. Thus, during the moderate decade, many Spanish physicians were drawn toward theorists who rejected the materialism and organicism of these psychologies in favor of a model of mental life based on an immortal, immaterial soul that vouchsafed free will and moral accountability.

Such reactions against the implications of materialist psychology were in keeping with the reactionary political mood that characterized Europe after 1815. As Edward Reed has detailed, throughout Europe during the first half of the nineteenth century there was a turn toward "traditional metaphysics," a dualistic faculty psychology that posited a disembodied mind comprising the emotions (or "sensibility"), the intellect, and the will. These three faculties existed in a hierarchy in which the intellect, by means of the will, exercised control over the emotions.[2] Traditional metaphysics drew on Immanuel Kant's dismissal of psychology as a natural science, echoing his skepticism of any necessary causal connection between external matter in motion and internal mental states.[3]

Chief among the traditional metaphysicians was Victor Cousin, the French philosopher whose "eclectic" psychology enjoyed an enormous influence in both Europe and America. While Cousin claimed his eclecticism had integrated the best that all previous systems had to offer, in reality his psychology misconstrued the findings of his sources and in the final analysis amounted to a thoroughgoing spiritualism in which self-consciousness was fully independent of the physiological processes of the body, and in which a mysterious and ill-defined faculty of "intuition" purported to provide direct access to the theological truths of religion.[4] The "militant spiritualism"—as Enric Novella has described it—of Cousinian traditional metaphysics was thoroughly institutionalized in Spain, as we can see in an 1850 dictate for Spanish institutes of education: "The professor of the class must provide a definition of psychology that carefully delineates the existence of the soul, its status as a substance distinct from matter and the human body, its attributes of unity, identity, and activity, and the primary and irreducible faculties of the human SELF: sensibility, intelligence, and will."[5] In a number of works, Novella has convincingly shown how the thoroughgoing spiritualism reflected in the preceding passage lay at the core of a bourgeois "politics of the self" that permeated mid-nineteenth-century Spanish culture.[6]

Throughout Europe, in the wake of the Congress of Vienna, questioning this vision of the self, and the traditional metaphysics underlying it, could be a dangerous endeavor, as evidenced by the fate of British physician William Lawrence. Lawrence insisted on a purely naturalistic approach to understanding mental phenomena, and in keeping with such an approach took up the question of mental illness and whether it was a physiological disorder rather than a spiritual one. For Lawrence, madness was unquestionably a physical impairment, and as such, curable through the ministrations of physicians. Rather than celebrating this fact, however, the British medical establishment declared Lawrence a heretic and forced him to recant.[7]

Surprisingly, given the repressive atmosphere elsewhere in Europe, Martínez participated in a remarkably wide-ranging discussion of issues surrounding the materiality of the mind and the etiology of mental illness. One forum for this discussion seems to have been the society founded by Martínez, the Medico-Surgical Society for Emulation and Reciprocal Instruction. Among Martínez's collected papers exists a transcript of an address read before the society on January 18, 1840, by a colleague of Martínez's, Bartolomé Alcalá y Pavón, who was one of the society's charter members. The address, copied by Martínez himself, was entitled "Fenómenos de la naturaleza" (Phenomena of Nature), and it argued for a thoroughly materialistic understanding of the mind.

Alcalá's presentation systematically dismantles arguments for an immaterial soul. He begins with a genealogy of the soul going back to Plato, who, according to Alcalá, was convinced that the body was "composed of two parts, one material and the other spiritual." Alcalá then describes how this Platonic dualism was adopted by the Church Fathers, who interpreted the soul as "an immediate emanation of the divine," an interpretation that became dominant going forward. This interpretation held that the soul "was an immaterial substance, eminently active, immortal, and imbued with the faculties of thought and desire."[8] Man, endowed with this immaterial soul, was judged to be the "essential being of the creation, and the only being capable of freely discerning and judging. Animals, in contrast were considered crude machines, without the faculty of judgment, and whose movements were governed by blind, immutable destiny. Such were the ideas that reigned supreme for almost two thousand years in all the nations of the civilized world."[9]

After surveying the origins of the spiritualist conception of the soul, Alcalá stakes out his own position: "In the first place, I will say to you that I am a pure materialist; that I consider imaginary all spiritual entities claimed to exist by the metaphysicians; that I consider all religions false and founded only on the vested interests of their ministers . . . ; that I consider the Christian religion to be an absurdity and one that above all reveals the spirit of avarice of its ministers."[10] After this polemical prolegomena, Alcalá promises to leave political and religious considerations aside, as "they are not part of the subject that concerns us here," and to "speak exclusively of that mysterious being—spiritual, indivisible, immaterial—that is thought to inhabit our body."[11] Alcalá then raises a pair of objections to the spiritualist position:

First of all, if we consider metaphysically the existence of the soul, we will see that it is imaginary; if this were not the case, then where would we receive knowledge of its existence? Just because we are ignorant of the mechanisms of the brain in certain acts of the intellect, is that reason enough to posit [the soul's] existence? No gentlemen, because in that case we could follow Bacon in positing a "sensible soul" just because we are ignorant of the mechanism of the nerves in acts of sensation; in other words, we could then posit as many souls in the body as there are functions that we cannot explain, which is an absurdity.

Secondly, I would ask those who posit the existence of the soul, how can we posit a thing without parts? How can such a thing exist and occupy a mathematical point? Well, gentlemen, I cannot comprehend how the existence of a thing can be compatible with a lack of parts and the failure to occupy space. In my opinion this means that it does not exist. It is impossible to measure a spiritual entity that has properties distinct from material bodies. The question then becomes, where, and by what means, could we measure these properties? Nature has endowed us with certain sense perceptions, both internal and external, so that we can enter into relation with the objects that surround us, so that we can study their positive and negative qualities, in order to satisfy our needs. . . . [We] can only have ideas of material things, and we can only reason accurately about such material things. . . . And thus leaving aside all metaphysical considerations, I will now examine the question physiologically, which is the proper means of resolving it.[12]

In restricting his investigations to the sphere of physiology, Alcalá lays his cards on the table, declaring that "the brain is not a single organ but rather composed of multiple organs which are responsible for exercising the various intellectual faculties, and this leaves two possibilities: either the soul is divided into various parts in order to preside over the different parts of the brain, or there are as many different souls as there are distinct parts of the brain."[13] He then concludes that, if we accept the first proposition, then the soul is divisible and hence material, and if we accept the second, then these souls must have separate natures and hence form a composite, heterogenous body, in which case we are dealing with a material entity; or in the case that these souls share the same nature, they would form a homogenous body, but still a material one.[14]

Despite his promise to avoid theological matters, Alcalá returns to the issue of religion in his conclusion, asserting that if religion is based on an erroneous claim—that is, the existence of an immaterial, immortal soul—then religion must be false. This does not mean, however, that religion serves no social function. On the contrary, "religious institutions have formed the basis for all civilizations," writes Alcalá, giving men hope for a better future in the next world and instilling in them a healthy fear of authority. "The founding legislators," he continues, "have always appeared to be divinely inspired and have spoken in the language of the divine to their contemporaries and imposed moral laws derived from this divine authority."[15] But while religion may have an instrumental value, when it comes to the nature of mind, Alcalá's professed goal is to provide "a solid and inalterable foundation, to form an exact and complete understanding of the most noble and sublime function of our machine."[16]

An Enlightened Eclecticism

Martínez took a keen interest in materialism, as evidenced by the painstaking, handwritten copy of Alcalá's dissertation that he made. Throughout his writings he expressed an appreciation of, and a tolerance toward, materialist conceptions, denying that they should be shunned as irreligious or subversive. He held that "materialism is a system like any other, and its proponents should be respected whatever their faith, as long as it is sincere."[17] Martínez was well-versed in the works of Ideologues such as Cabanis, and phrenologists such as Gall and Spurzheim, and he also made reference to Erasmus Darwin's *Zoonomia* in his writings.[18] But despite his sympathy toward the materialist position, Martínez was not willing to embrace the atheism of his colleague Alcalá; he sought instead to formulate what he called an "enlightened eclecticism" that would combat the mainstream eclecticism of Cousin and his ilk, which he dismissed as a "disguised spiritualism."[19] Central to this task was an early modern Spanish tradition of organicist theorizing on the soul that Martínez drew upon in order to provide an alternative account that would preserve a place for religious truth, while also being compatible with the organicism of contemporary nineteenth-century theorists. This account had the added benefit of highlighting heroes of la medicina patria.

In the sixteenth century, Spanish theorists pioneered a naturalizing approach to the study of the relationship between soul and soma, an approach epitomized by the works of figures such as Gomez Pereira, Oliva Sabuco, and Juan Huarte. These thinkers all shared an emphasis on the physiological basis of psychic phenomena and championed a cerebrocentrism that posited the brain as the essential organ of human thought. Perhaps the most radical of the three was Pereira, whose *Antoniana Margarita* (1554) presented a mechanistic model of the brain that came to be seen as having anticipated the work of Descartes and later developments in neuroscience concerning the electrical conduction of nerve impulses.[20] But the two most important contributors to Martínez's medico-political project were Huarte and Sabuco, both of whom posited an intimate, reciprocal, and inescapable relationship between soul and body, one which determined everything from the vicissitudes of physical and mental health to the formation of enduring personality traits.

Like Pereira, Huarte and Sabuco have been regularly touted as harbingers of later developments in the history of medicine. They have been associated, for example, with a "Renaissance organicism" that anticipated subsequent vitalist concepts, and their doctrines have even been compared to the psychoanalysis of Sigmund Freud.[21] My goal, however, is not to provide yet another analysis of these currents and connections in an attempt to discern the definitive intellectual influences at play; my interest here is not so much the history of medicine as the history of medico-political discourse. In familiar Renaissance fashion, Huarte and Sabuco tailored a variety of classical sources—from Plato and Aristotle to Hippocrates and Galen—to fit their own medico-political moment.[22] Likewise, Martínez made use of the works of Huarte and Sabuco during the liberal revolution of the nineteenth century to advance his own medico-political agenda.

Martínez's first writings on Huarte were undertaken in his 1842 dissertation, wherein he compares Huarte's doctrines concerning the brain to those of contemporary nineteenth-century researchers. In the dissertation, Martínez declares that since antiquity it has been accepted that the moral determines the physical, and the body was seen to be a servant of the soul, "the one obeying the other like a tyrant and a slave."[23] In the present day, Martínez continues, it is generally accepted that the body modifies the soul, but there has been a tendency to go to the opposite extreme in postulating a thoroughgoing somatic determinism. Indeed, many eighteenth- and nineteenth-century theorists had put forth elaborate systems seeking to link personality traits and moral attributes to anatomical structures. Martínez mentions the physiognomy of the Swiss philosopher and theologian Johann Kaspar Lavater, only to dismiss it as "fanatical and lacking proof."[24] More promising, according to Martínez, was the work of the German physician-scientist Franz Joseph Gall, whose research into the localization of brain function sought to determine the brain's role in generating individual aptitudes, much in the same manner as Huarte.[25] In Martínez's opinion, however, Gall was carried away by unfounded speculations concerning the craneoscope, an instrument that was thought to be able to measure protuberances in the skull, and thereby identify aspects of brain structure that could account for various traits and aptitudes. Martínez points out that Huarte predicted many elements of Gall's system, and as a result has been recognized as an important contributor to medical science: "The work of this wise fellow countryman was epochal not only in the history of Spanish medicine, but in the history of European medicine as well, and as such it has been appreciated by wise men who recognize the merit of this distinguished Spaniard."[26] Martínez insists that Huarte's achievement is even more heroic, given that it was accomplished during a period in which he could not express himself freely due to religious strictures that forced him to resort to "many circumlocutions" when it came to sensitive theological issues.[27]

Oliva Sabuco's approach to the mind-body problem was similarly controversial. Sabuco's principle theses were (1) that the brain is the central organ of the human body, responsible for directing all physical and spiritual functions through the dispersal of a cerebrospinal fluid, or "nervous juice," or "*chilo*," and (2) that the passions are the organic cause of disease.[28] These assertions garnered suspicion not only from the Church, but from the medical establishment as well. Contrary to Galenic orthodoxy, which insisted that health consisted of a balance of the humors, Sabuco argued that the health of the body is determined through the interaction between the stomach, which is hot and dry, and the brain, which is cool and moist. In this temperature differential lies the root of illness, and this differential is regulated by the passions, located in the brain.[29] The centrality of the brain in Sabuco's schema deviated from earlier paradigms which focused on the heart, or the liver, as the nutritive organs of the body; for Sabuco, it was instead the aforementioned nervous juice, derived from the brain's moisture, that nourished the body, spreading as if it were an inverted tree with the brain as its root, sending the vital fluid to the leaves and branches.[30] As Sabuco put it: "The brain is the cause and workshop of all diseases' humors. There, in the brain, reside the feelings, passions, and motions of the soul; there is the seat of sense perception; there is the root."[31] The distribution and quality of the nervous juice could be affected by the passions, and thus Sabuco's system was a psychosomatic one in which mental and emotional states impacted the health of the body, or to quote Sabuco once again, "The main cause of bad juice is the spiritual passions, which are peculiar to man, and this is why man has so many diseases that the other animals do not have."[32]

The emphasis here on the passions resonated with nineteenth-century treatments, and just as he compared Huarte to Gall, in his new edition of *La nueva filosofía*, Martínez ranked Sabuco's work in relation to contemporary treatises, such as Alibert's *Physiologie des passions*: "If we consider the matter calmly and reflectively, that Alibert—an erudite man and facile writer without a doubt—composed his work two hundred years after our Oliva, it is amazing that the Frenchman has not improved on the distinguished Spanish doctor."[33] Martínez was not the only one to compare Sabuco to Alibert; Juan Mosácula, in his treatise on human physiology, made a similar comparison, as did Félix Janer in several articles published in the *Gaceta Médica de Madrid* (*Medical Gazette of Madrid*).[34] Antonio Hernández Morejón and Anastasio Chinchilla Piqueras also wrote biobibliographical sketches of both Huarte and Sabuco and drew comparisons between their doctrines and contemporary medical theories.

Chinchilla even dabbled in the popular conversation concerning the relationship between the physical and the moral. In a speech presented at the inaugural session of the Academia Médico-Quirújica de Castilla la Nueva (the Medico-Surgical Academy of New Castile), and later published in the *Boletín del Instituto Médico Valenciano* (*Bulletin of the Medical Institute of Valencia*), Chinchilla held forth on the "moral system" of man, which he considered to be "the very perfection of the order of creation."[35] This moral system, in typical spiritualist fashion, depended on a disembodied soul as the guarantor of free will and access to religious truth, a position very much in keeping with the bourgeois "politics of the self" detailed in the previous section. According to Chinchilla,

> The Creator delegated to man a part of his dominion over the earth; He created a noble, sublime creature, somehow capable of uniting heaven and earth. For such an exalted destiny, it was necessary to distinguish this noble endeavor from organized matter by means of an infusion of His faculties. In this way He made man free; if it had been otherwise, it would have been nothing more than modifying a bit of matter, as in the case of brute animals. He presented to man the idea of good and evil, justice and injustice, and said to him: *you are free.*[36]

Chinchilla then went on to emphasize how this moral freedom depended, predictably, on a stark dualism between soul and body, on a "thinking spirit which is the depository of our knowledge of good and evil." And this "thinking spirit" equated to the soul, or self: "This is our soul, this is the *self* that reasons, the *self* through which we are able to comprehend in a single instant all the parts of the earth without moving an inch, this is the *self* that commands the body, and which the body obeys."[37]

Whereas other writers may have composed brief biographies of Sabuco and Huarte and provided summaries of their works, and may have even speculated on the relationship between the "physical and the moral," Martínez, in contrast, endeavored to enlist these early modern luminaries in a much larger and more ambitious medico-political project. The figures of Juan Huarte de San Juan and Oliva Sabuco de Nantes served several purposes for Martínez: they functioned as heroes of la medicina patria and examples of what Spanish medicine was capable of; they could also be construed as medical martyrs by virtue of having been censored by the Inquisition, and thereby serve as testaments to the backwardness of the old regime; finally, and most significantly, their organicist models of brain function which emphasized the physiology of the passions and the genesis of personality types (that is, the relationship between the physical and the moral) made them especially valuable resources for Martínez as he endeavored to mediate between early modern Spanish medico-political literature and the nineteenth-century science of man.

In his 1847 commentary on Sabuco's *Nueva filosofía*, Martínez outlined his strategy, writing, "It is undeniable that if we follow the principles of philosophy with complete liberty, it seems to me that we arrive at a middle way: the path of an enlightened eclecticism."[38] Martínez sought to chart a course between the Scylla of a materialism that reduced "man to the condition of an animal" and the Charybdis of a spiritualism that "sings to the heavens the praises of spiritual man, raising him to the status of the angels." In reality, however, this middle way was not equally poised between spiritualism and materialism, as Martínez repeatedly insisted that materialism must be given its due, asserting, for example, that the materialist position was "more logical than the opposing one."[39]

The spiritualists, according to Martínez, posited a "who-knows-what," an active, spiritual principle "born of the Supreme Being as a divine emanation, a special particle in which reside the faculties of reason and thought. These faculties are immaterial, just like the cause that produces them, and they cannot be modified by the body except in an accidental and accessory manner. . . . [I]t is independent from the organism in its action, and it is imperishable and immortal. . . . Those who defend this doctrine see the body as passive, always subject to a well-organized soul."[40] The spiritualist position characterized here is similar to the doctrines of Spanish eclectics such as Monlau, whose descriptions of the relationship between body and soul portrayed the soul as an active force acting upon a passive body: "The life of the soul is a life that knows itself, an autonomous force that is self-directed and is conscious of its own energy and faculties; it is an independent cause, a *vita sui conscia, sui potens, sui motrix*. . . . Physical forces are automatic; psychic forces are autocratic."[41] Martínez, in contrast, postulated the existence of a force that "operates and executes, and is manifested in concert with the corporeal and material organs."[42] This is a force that cannot be demonstrated through reason or the senses; it can only be inferred from the "intimacy of self-consciousness," and we are unable to "demonstrate the qualities with which it is adorned, and even less so its nature. Thus, it can be deduced that we only know of its existence through its exterior manifestations, and these

exterior manifestations form what we must denote as its laws."[43] In keeping
with the early modern theorizing of Huarte and Sabuco, Martínez's brand of
eclecticism posited a reciprocal relationship between soul and soma in which
the organs of the body function as instruments through which the soul's directives are carried out: "Now, it is undeniable that, whatever its nature, [the
soul] needs the organs of the body as instruments, which it commands and
directs in a certain fashion, and to the degree to which these instruments are
perfected, the better they are able to fulfill the commands of the soul."[44] In
other words, because in this model all souls are of equal perfection, any difference in ability must be a result of a difference in the material composition
of the body, and thus the bodily organs played an active role in the exercise
of the powers of the soul.

Martínez, then, put forward a schema in which body and soul were not
in conflict with one another. Rather than a battle between the spirit and the
flesh, his "enlightened eclecticism" envisioned mind and matter in a continuous, harmonious exchange:

> As it is beyond doubt that the soul, as an active principle, modifies and
> determines the will and actions when the organism is functioning harmo-
> niously; likewise, the body modifies the conditions of the soul by means of
> external sensations that determine it, that force [the soul] in a certain way;
> from here we conclude that the body is also an active principle in relation
> with external objects, which modifies the soul, and consequently, man is
> composed of two active principles, the body and the soul—two currents,
> one internal or centrifugal, which is the soul, the other external or centrip-
> etal, which is the body, and both of these mutually modify one another.[45]

For Martínez, this amounted to "the true eclecticism," which he likened to
Stahl's animism, wherein the soul is a "power that combines and disposes,
while the organs work as instruments under its direction."[46]

Martínez's invocation of Georg Ernst Stahl is significant, since Stahl's
doctrine has been put forth as a precursor to the vitalist theories that were
a fixture of the mid-nineteenth-century medico-political milieu. Stahl postulated the soul as a sort of "physiological propeller," a force that used the
body as an *organon,* vivifying it over and above its material substrate.[47] The
extent to which Stahl's conception of the soul was in keeping with Sabuco

and Huarte's views is open to debate; their early modern formulations, while often critical of Aristotle and Galen, were nevertheless by and large within the Aristotelian-Galenic paradigm, and they construed the soul as intrinsically embodied.[48] Stahl, in contrast, posited the soul as something immaterial and external to inert matter, a principle that is added to the body as a means of vivifying it and thereby staving off corruption and decay.[49] Putting aside questions concerning the accuracy of Martínez's proposed parallel, it is no wonder that he made this connection, seeing as his project was to establish the contemporary relevance of Sabuco and Huarte, and while the animism of Stahl was perhaps not a vitalism per se, it was celebrated by later vitalists as a crucial rebuttal to mechanism and as a powerful argument for the existence of a vital force in nature.[50]

Vitalism was a hot topic in Spain as elsewhere, and Martínez took up the issue in his 1840 dissertation, wherein he warned his colleagues against the excesses of vitalist theorizing:

> Fanatical mortals, stop enquiring after first causes and essences—study only the effects; observe, experiment, interrogate nature with modesty, and thus shall you advance your investigations! In effect, gentlemen, have we advanced physiology more with the invention of a "vital principle" and the deliriums of Paracelsus than through the observation and practice of Galen and Hippocrates? Certainly not; rather we have set back our knowledge of effects that are clearly due to alterations in the [corporeal] organization, attributing them instead to this particular principle, which is sometimes considered a form of intelligence, and other times no, and which serves above all to manifest our insufficiency. We use the word as if it meant that we actually know something, but in resorting to this explanation we only prove our own ignorance. . . . The word "vital" is how we doctors describe something that we do not understand, like the physicists with their "attraction," and the chemists with their "affinity."[51]

While at first glance Martínez's diatribe may seem to be a rejection of vitalism, it was actually a common rhetorical stance among nineteenth-century vitalist physicians. For example, the renowned Montpellier vitalist Paul-Joseph Barthez repeatedly declared himself a proponent of Baconian empiricism and cautioned against reifying the vital principle, or taking it as an "explanation of phenomena" rather than a "necessary abstraction,"[52] and François-Joseph-Victor Broussais harshly criticized vitalism, yet he availed himself of vitalist conceptions and vocabulary; indeed, his celebrated doctrine of "irritability" could be seen as approximating vitalist constructs. So it is, in fact, not necessarily contradictory that Martínez should rail against vitalism and then go on to admit the need for some sort of vital principle to make sense of living beings: "I understand that life is an effect, and that all effects entail a cause, and that in the interest of clarity it is necessary to give it a name: consequently, I accept the existence of a cause that produces life (a vital principle) and through the process of generation imbues a general property to all organic beings."[53] In his "Treatise on Physiology," Martínez reluctantly offers another, somewhat tautological, defense of vitalism: "Unable to see any alternative, we accept the system of the vitalists; because it is very certain that the vital phenomena cannot be explained in any other way, since it is impossible for physical and chemical forces to become vitalized without uniting with other elements in such a state. For this reason we must exclude all theories that seek to explain the phenomena of life by resorting exclusively to physical and chemical laws without taking into account the laws of vital force."[54]

It could be argued that some sort of vitalist notion is necessary to the organicist psychosomaticism of Sabuco and Huarte. Their insistence on a reciprocal, organic relationship between soul and body allowed a much greater role for material causation than was typical for the time (hence, the suspicion on the part of the religious authorities), but there had to remain an immaterial aspect—or at least something irreducible to the physico-chemical laws of nature—to interact with the "instruments" of the human body. Of course, this version of organicism contrasts with nineteenth-century organicism, which defined itself over and against vitalism in its insistence that every disease could be traced to a specific organic lesion in the body. But in reality, these distinctions were in a constant state of flux during the period, and numerous historians of science have argued that the nineteenth-century organicists' style of materialism was in fact compatible with vitalism, insofar as the organic changes they linked to disease were only intelligible in the context of the structure and function of a living organism—which amounted to, in essence, a form of "vitalist materialism."[55]

The goal here is not to delve into what has aptly been described as the "bewildering variety of early nineteenth-century vitalisms,"[56] but rather to emphasize that Ildefonso Martínez did not neatly conform to the standard dichotomies that have been drawn between vitalism and materialism and their political correlates. José María López Piñero, for example, has asserted that moderado physicians tended toward older, vitalist theories, while progresistas championed mechanism, positivism, and experimentalism, but the case of Ildefonso Martínez highlights the complexities of the situation on the ground.[57] Martínez was unmistakably on the left with regard to his political orientation, but he was sympathetic to vitalism nonetheless, and when it came to experimentalism his position was ambiguous.

The characterization of vitalism as politically conservative and scientifically retrograde has a long history and was epitomized in the mid-nineteenth-century Great Debate on Hippocrates, in which the prominent physician Pedro Mata y Fontanet took aim at neo-Hippocratic vitalism and its supporters in the Spanish medical establishment, such as Matías Nieto y Serrano.[58] Mata, an associate of Martínez's in several professional organizations and a contributor to his newspaper, *El Crisol*,[59] lambasted vitalism not merely as a scientific theory, but as a proxy for everything he detested about the conservative moderado status quo that he felt was retarding Spain's modernization, medically as well as politically. The irony here, as Nicolás Fernández-Medina has observed, is that Mata's excoriation of Spain's backwardness was not buttressed by forward-looking references to cutting-edge positivist materialism, but rather by invocations of ancient authority. Just as Ildefonso Martínez advocated for his enlightened eclecticism by looking backward to heroes of la medicina patria, such as Huarte and Sabuco, Mata looked to the atomists of ancient Greece, such as Anaximander, Heraclitus, and Democritus.[60] And to complicate matters further still, Fernández-Medina argues persuasively that—contrary to Mata's critique—vitalism was not a relic of the past, but rather an important aspect of Spanish modernity: "What Mata y Fontanet could not see with clarity was the extent to which vitalist theories were being assimilated and reinterpreted through the emerging discourses of evolutionism, hygiene, calisthenics, homeopathy, and psychology, discourses that would fundamentally modernize culture and science across Spain and Europe in a few short years."[61]

When it comes to providing evidence of skepticism concerning the experimental method, López Piñero quotes an article from Ildefonso Martínez's decidedly progressive publication, *El Crisol,* as an example of anti-experimentalism.[62] López Piñero cites a profile that appeared in the periodical denouncing physician Joaquín Hysern for "giving a great deal of importance to experiments."[63] It is not entirely clear whether this represented a wholesale rejection of experimentation, however. The chief complaint seems to have been with Hysern's pedagogical approach, which digressed into discussions of experimentation at the expense of material that had to be covered in order to meet the requirements for the degree. Elsewhere, Martínez criticized Hysern for *neglecting* the importance of experimentation. Hysern was a star in the Spanish medical firmament; he had studied with the celebrated physiologist Magendie in France, and on his return to Spain he became a leading proponent of homeopathy, which had attracted numerous adherents, but also many critics. One of these critics was Ildefonso Martínez, who heaped scorn on the homeopaths in a treatise titled "Homeopato-mania."[64] Writing under the pseudonym Doctor Barlo-Vento," Martínez excoriated physicians such as Hysern for their embrace of homeopathy precisely because it was not supported by experimental evidence.[65]

Given the complexities involved in pinning down Martínez's precise medical ideology, when it comes to assessing his "enlightened eclecticism" I will not attempt to characterize it in relation to some idealized taxonomy of scientific thought, but rather seek to understand how it was used as a rhetorical strategy in the medico-political environment of mid-nineteenth-century Spain. Like the spiritualized version of eclecticism he sought to combat, Martínez's enlightened eclecticism was labile and capable of being deployed in a variety of ways. Just as Victor Cousin played fast and loose with his philosophical forbears, Martínez deployed his cadre of Spanish Renaissance natural philosophers with different emphases according to the situation.

The pliability of Martínez's strategy is evident in his response to the French physician and churchman Abbé Laurent Cerise, whose spiritualist eclecticism had put him at odds with both Gall and Huarte. In his *Exposé et examen critique du système phrénologique* (*Exposé and Critical Examination of the System of Phrenology*), Cerise singled out Huarte as a precursor to the materialism of Gall and the phrenologists, and went on to assert that Huarte's doctrines conflicted with Catholic orthodoxy, as they represented "one of a thousand examples of the materialist consequences logically derived from a false science."[66] In response, Martínez suggested that Cerise was "too much of a spiritualist" and claimed that he had misconstrued Huarte's ideas, which were in fact compatible with the teachings of the Church. It is indeed the case that, while scholars have long emphasized Huarte's heterodox views and have highlighted his materialist tendencies, in the *Examen* Huarte provides an extended argument for the immortality of the soul in an attempt to reconcile his psychological system with Catholic doctrine.

In a recent article Ismael del Olmo has described these maneuvers, explaining how after thoroughly naturalizing and medicalizing the phenomenon of diabolism, Huarte dedicates chapter 7 of the *Examen* to a proof of the immortality of the soul, using demonic possession as an analogy.[67] Huarte argues, citing many examples from Scripture, that demons are only able to inhabit a human body when its physical disposition is amenable, and when this disposition deteriorates, demons flee, without themselves deteriorating.[68] Huarte then proceeds to draw a parallel with the rational soul, which having "the same nature as demons and angels" likewise requires the appropriate physical conditions to inhabit a human body: "In order to operate, the rational soul and the devil avail themselves of material qualities, and some of these repulse and others attract. For this reason they are drawn to certain places and flee from others, without being corruptible themselves."[69] Such a view was not necessarily incompatible with Huarte's naturalism. For example, an overabundance of the melancholic humor was, for Huarte, one of the physical conditions that facilitated demonic possession, and thus a physician could treat such an imbalance of the humors and thereby expel demons without any need for a priest.

Cerise was familiar with Huarte's demonological analogy and referenced it disapprovingly in his *Exposé:* "Huarte and his contemporaries, in their naive faith, had come to accept a science that was far from being in accord with [Catholic doctrine]: and this contradiction proved to be a constant embarrassment. The doctor went so far as to ask himself if the influence of the devil, which causes evil inclinations, can function in man without taking advantage of the bad corporeal qualities in which he likes to reside; and if the acts of God can produce good inclinations without the support of the good corporeal qualities in which he delights."[70] Martínez, after quoting Cerise's criticism of Huarte, sought to turn the tables, insisting that Huarte's proof of an immaterial soul was actually compatible with the position of Cerise—that it was, in fact, "impossible to express more clearly or simply the eclecticism of the present day."[71] Martínez pointed out that, despite his avowed spiritualism, Cerise conceded that the soul must operate through corporeal instruments: "But if we take into account that Cerise is too much of a spiritualist, and that he himself says man comprises an active spirit which commands the passive flesh, without which he can do nothing, it is easy to see that he is being inconsistent in his attack on Huarte, since Huarte is saying the same thing as Cerise, only in different words; he repeats many times that in order for the soul to operate it must use the organs of the body as instruments."[72] Granted, this was somewhat disingenuous. Martínez's "enlightened eclecticism" was not based on the idea of purely passive matter being animated by an immaterial soul; rather, it gave pride of place to the ideas of Huarte and Sabuco precisely because they posited a more dynamic, reciprocal relationship between mind and matter than would have been acceptable to Cerise and his fellow eclectics. As Cerise made clear, while the soul might operate via "carnal instruments," in his psychology it was a strictly unidirectional causation, far from the "flagrant materialism" of the phrenologists: "Man is an activity that manifests itself through carnal instruments. The source of this activity could not be in these instruments themselves which never move spontaneously, which need to be excited to be moved, whose character is an absolute passivity. This affirmation is rigorously true, psychologically and physiologically. Phrenology, on the contrary, proclaims that the activity of the organs is the source of all the determinations and of all the moral and intellectual operations of man."[73]

This was, to be sure, a tendentious characterization of Gall's phrenology, but a familiar one. Charges of materialism, many of them politically motivated, had been leveled against Gall going back to his time in Vienna, when he was singled out by the Emperor Francis II and forbidden from lecturing in the midst of the politically charged period of the Napoleonic Wars.[74] Whatever one's position vis-à-vis the dangers of materialism, suffice it to say that merely asserting that the soul required instruments in the form of organs in order to function in the human body was unlikely to co-opt spiritualists like Cerise, or anyone else, for that matter. Such an assertion amounted to little more than a truism in the mid-nineteenth century; it was compatible with the position taken by the militant spiritualists, but also with the position of positivists such as Pedro Mata, who wrote: "The powers of the soul cannot manifest themselves without organs, and all organic activity is functional; thus, it falls under the dominion and jurisdiction of physiology. All psychology that is not functional or physiological is completely false."[75] Without clearly specifying the precise nature of the instruments and their relationship to the soul (or lack thereof), there was little to be gained by merely invoking a physiological nexus between psyche and soma. When it came to such assertions in the realm of mid-nineteenth-century medicine, the devil was quite literally in the details.

Medicine and Madness

The various eclecticisms circulating during the period were by their very nature geared toward presenting an image of reasonableness between extremes rather than a rigorously coherent set of scientific principles, and Martínez's "enlightened eclecticism" was no exception. The inherent malleability of the eclectic stance made it possible for Martínez to attempt to co-opt the spiritual eclecticism of Cerise and Cousin, and then do an about face in order to wield the heroes of la medicina patria against what he perceived to be the spiritualist obscurantism of the medical moderados. We can see this strategy at work in the contentious debate surrounding the etiology of mental illness in nineteenth-century Spain, wherein Martínez mobilized the Renaissance organicism of Huarte and Sabuco in support of the organicism of the physicians of the "French school," which had sought to naturalize insanity as the product of physical lesions in the brain. In so doing, Martínez characteristically sought to position himself between extremes; on the one hand, he reminded his readers, "We do not give much credit to spiritualism, and we have struggled to avoid returning to the days when medicine could only say of mental afflictions: 'the diseases of the soul are not our concern; we treat them only as moral problems,'" and insisted that "the more we study physiology, the more we will advance in pathology."[76] On the other hand, he adopted this robust somaticism without asserting an extreme localization of function, insisting on the folly of attributing "every function or action to a specific organ," a position he took to be "an abstraction born out of belief and dogma."[77]

Mental illness was a shared preoccupation for sixteenth-century medico-political theorists and the nineteenth-century science of man. The drive on the part of Huarte and Sabuco to correlate structures and functions of the brain with specific moral virtues, aptitudes, and abilities invited speculation regarding how these processes might go awry. Likewise, the "science of ideas" which had animated the French Ideologues, with its intense focus on the mind-body relationship, inevitably led to an interest in mental illness. Indeed, the period in which the Ideologues were active has been characterized as "the golden age of alienism."[78] It was during this time that George Cabanis himself, while serving as the director of Paris hospitals, hired Philippe Pinel, who famously removed the chains from the inmates at Bicêtre and the Salpêtrière, thereby inaugurating the age of modern psychiatry. As a partisan of the science of man, Pinel recognized the influence of the physical on the moral, and vice versa, and consequently advocated the "moral treatment" of mental illness—which is to say, the practice of psychotherapy—an approach that posited a reciprocal relationship between the psychological and the physiological.[79] Predictably, Ildefonso Martínez approved of Pinel's approach and argued that it had been anticipated in the ideas of Huarte and Sabuco.

Debates over the causes of insanity inevitably took on a political dimension in the nineteenth century. Observers across the political spectrum agreed that the ever-increasing pace of political and technological change was responsible for a dramatic upsurge in mental illness. This agreement dissipated quickly, however, when it came to diagnosing precisely which changes were to blame. Conservatives typically found fault with the advent of democracy, a charge that Martínez undertook to counter in an article in *El Crisol*. Martínez rejected the idea that representative governments are more likely to cause mental disorders and insisted instead that despotic governments "exert a great influence on their subjects and produce many mental illnesses, especially suicides, as we see with the demise of liberty in ancient Rome, which resulted in a multitude of suicides and mad men and women under the reigns of Tiberius, Caligula, and other tyrannical emperors."[80] Martínez admits that more advanced countries sometimes record higher levels of insanity, but attributes this to their more efficient methods of collecting data. Also, these more advanced countries do more to treat mental illnesses by providing asylums and medical care, rather than leaving the insane to their own devices. Democratic governments, according to Martínez, far from fomenting mental illness, do more to assuage it, unlike the "partisans of the old regime who wage eternal war against reform."[81]

Martínez's interest in mental illness led him to submit a proposal for reforming the treatment of the mentally ill in Spain. Addressing himself to

"Her Majesty's government," Martínez advocated a thorough reform of the system of mental health care as a means of bringing Spain in line with what was being done in "the more civilized countries of Europe." He prefaces the proposal with a description of the sorry state of affairs in Spain, noting that there are precious few Spanish authors who deal with the topic of mental illness, and conceding that "we are very backwards in this branch of knowledge compared with other, happier nations."[82] As in his newspaper article, Martínez links madness to political upheaval, asking rhetorically, "do not political revolts produce the greater part of mental breakdowns? Let us not give way to the passions, but rather let reason speak, search the annals of history of the human race and you will find hair-raising examples of this truth."[83] Focusing his analysis on contemporary Spain, Martínez denounces the rank partisanship characterizing Spanish society while also taking a shot at one of his favorite targets, religious fanaticism: "The fire of revolution has yet to be extinguished, religious fanaticism has been revived; this mixture, this agitated confusion of ideas and conflicting doctrines, these are the elements most conducive to the production of mental illness."[84] Spain's problems derived, according to Martínez, from the outmoded, purely spiritualist approach to mental illness, and the solution lay in supplementing this approach with the teachings of the "organicist" school in an effort to explore the reciprocal relationship between mind and body: "[T]here are very few in Spain who have dedicated themselves to the difficult study of man as a duality of body and spirit, who appears on the one hand as an animal and on the other as a rational being; one thing is certain: there has been no attempt on our part to marry the principles of the school of Plato, Kant, Leibnitz, Malebranche, Descartes, and the philosophers of the spiritualist school with that of Locke, Condillac, Destutt de Tracy, Cabanis, and Broussais, that is to say the organicist school."[85]

This organicist understanding of mental functions was politically fraught. The orthodox position was decidedly spiritualist, as evidenced by the writings of Matías Nieto y Serrano.[86] Nieto was a fixture in the medico-political debates of mid-century Spain, and was one of the founders of the conservative moderado medical periodical *El Siglo Médico*. Nieto was also the quintessential traditional metaphysician, having been greatly influenced by German idealism in general, and Kant in particular. He was implacably hostile toward any attempt to naturalize the cognitive faculties or associate mental disorders with specific lesions to the brain. He composed a series of diatribes in the pages of *El Siglo Médico* decrying such efforts and denouncing the "band of organicists of the Parisian school" and their attempts to establish "a necessary causal relationship between the diverse classes of phenomena displayed by the human organism, between the structure of the brain, for example, and the intellectual and affective activities."[87] Endeavoring to summarize the controversy, Nieto wrote: "In short, it is about establishing whether a little bit of hardness or softness, ruddiness or pallor, or a little more or less blood in the brain, or visible, tangible, lesions found in a cadaver, can account for the disruption of the faculties of the soul that we refer to as madness; or whether a spirit, an immaterial thing functioning as the cause of life and reason independent of the bodily organs, is the cause of the material lesions that are sometimes found in the affected subjects."[88] Given these competing hypotheses, Nieto insisted there was no possible way to definitively rule out either one, which meant, in effect, that there could be no such thing as a scientific psychology that was able to diagnose and treat mental illness as a purely physiological disorder.

Faced with this skeptical position, Ildefonso Martínez sought to bring to bear his "enlightened eclecticism" on the etiology of mental illness. Whereas he had previously sought to show that the ideas of Huarte and Sabuco were compatible with the spiritualism of Cerise and the immortality of the soul, he was now determined to demonstrate that mental illness was an organic, rather than spiritual, phenomenon. In the case of Sabuco, Martínez, in his annotations to *La nueva filosofía*, highlighted her focus on the passions as the cause of mental disorders, with an attendant emphasis on the brain as the physiological nexus of such disorders. According to Sabuco, the origin of "every disease is the brain; therein are the passions, affects, and movements of the soul."[89] As we have seen, in the *Nueva filosofía* Sabuco offered a naturalistic account of mental illness based on the circulation of the "nerve juice," or *chilo*. The psychosomaticism of Sabuco's system accounts for the vicious cycle wherein destructive passions drain the energizing *chilo* from the brain, which in turn creates increasingly unhealthy emotional states. So, for example, "tedium and regret are more draining than other affections," and when this drainage becomes excessive, mental illness is the result: "Madness is the drainage of the *chilo* of the brain" and "from the same deficiency, i.e. the corruption of the brain, despair, sudden and difficult death, tedium, sadness, wrath, madness, rage, and all kinds of illnesses are due to the depression of the brain. [The exact medical condition that develops] depends on the extensiveness [of the drainage of brain fluid, humor, or *chilo*] and the region of the brain that is affected by it."[90]

Turning to the work of Juan Huarte, Martínez cited with approval his physiological localization of the passions and credited him with anticipating the work of contemporary theorists on mental illness: "Not only did Huarte seek to establish the location of the vices and virtues, but he also wished to undertake a therapeutic approach to the passions in order to cure them; it is a testament to his great genius that he accomplished the difficult study of the moral perturbations that has been advanced in recent times by the likes of Pinel and Esquirol."[91] In his *Examen,* Huarte had argued that the brain gives rise to the three discrete faculties of imagination, understanding, and memory, and that consequently, insanity could manifest itself solely in terms of one of these faculties without affecting the others.[92] Martínez cautioned that he was only proposing the ideas of Huarte as a hypothesis, but he hoped that they could serve as "a beacon" to guide further study: "We advance this only as a hypothesis, until we are convinced otherwise by deeper and more philosophical investigations, and it bears repeating that the difficult study of mental illnesses has only just begun; [at this point] it can be said to be merely empirical rather than philosophical, because physiology has not made sufficient progress when it comes to the moral and physical study of man."[93] Indeed, Martínez hoped to continue his work on Huarte in light of other contemporary medical issues, such as animal magnetism, if he were to be granted the "time and life" to do so.[94]

Having surveyed the status of the debate as to whether mental illness was a spiritual or physiological disorder in the light of the contributions of Huarte and Sabuco, Martínez concludes, "Insanity is a cerebral condition, usually chronic, without fever, and characterized by disorders of the sense perceptions, the intelligence, and the will."[95] The benefit to Martínez of the dynamic, reciprocal relationship between mind and matter posited by Sabuco and Huarte was that, while it emphasized the central role of the brain, it did not fall into what he considered to be the overly rigid localization of mental functions put forth by theorists such as Gall, and allowed for a unified, embodied self, but one that was "free from an exclusively organic monopoly,"[96] and could, consequently, ensure moral accountability. This enlightened eclectic position gave a nod to the orthodox eclectic focus on selfhood, but it contrasted with the strict mind-body dualism of the militant spiritualists in which an immaterial self functioned as the organizing principle of all interior phenomena and in which insanity was seen as a spiritual affliction.[97] But while in principle Martínez could claim to occupy the middle ground, being the ardent polemicist that he was, when push came to shove he persistently wielded his pen in favor of a markedly materialist conception of mental illness in the many debates that broke out in the Spanish medical press.

One such debate revolved around Félix García Caballero's treatise *De la libertad moral en sus relaciones con los delitos* (*On Free Will and Its Relationship with Crime*). García Caballero, a frequent contributor to the medical press, and to *El Siglo Médico* in particular, was a hard-and-fast spiritualist who dismissed the organicist conception of insanity and insisted on a radically dualistic conception of the human being in order to push back against those who would use mental illness as a way of mitigating moral and legal responsibility: "Man is, it appears, a composite of two substances: one immaterial, spiritual, intelligent, active, sensible, endowed with will and moral liberty—this is ordinarily called *soul* or *spirit;* the other is material by nature, incapable of thought or feeling—it is called *body*, which is organized matter, the result of divisible particles imbued with movement and life by an immaterial force, and thus subject to different laws, alterations, changes, destruction and death."[98] For García, this dualism is crucial to maintaining order and administering justice, as it underwrites man's free will and responsibility to society, virtues threatened by the theorizing of the organicists:

> The most prominent philosophers who believe in the omnipotence of the brain exclude *a fortiori* the existence of the soul, the human spirit as judge and ruler of all, the center of thought and of the sentiments that ennoble and divinize man, and instead imbue the brain with the power to dictate which actions are to be called good and evil, and consequently reduce man to the status of a menial and abject servant of his organization. . . . They claim that the soul does not exist, that perception, thought, judgment, memory, will, and the affections are all the immediate result of cerebral action, or better yet, modes of excitation of the nervous system, and that as a result, virtue and vice are consequences of the struggle between the encephalitic organ and the principal viscera, the modifications of which are perceived in the

sensorium and form the passions. What manifest errors! . . . What crude philosophizing! To make the nobility of human reason dependent on matter! There is no shortage of arguments against this philosophy of Hobbes, Spinoza, and their disciples Helvetius, Lamettrie, Gall, and Broussais, etc.[99]

These philosophers are mistaken in García's view because matter is incapable of thought; "there is as much distance between matter and thought," writes Garcia, "as between matter and the void."

García Caballero received a glowing notice in *El Siglo Médico*, wherein the reviewer wrote that, while it was "not a perfect work," the ideas it contained were of "great importance and truly momentous for the administration of justice."[100] The book received a quite different treatment in the pages of *El Crisol* in an article written under the pseudonym "la Avispa," (the Wasp). The author is unmistakably Martínez, as evidenced by the acid wit and repeated invocations of Juan Huarte. Reacting to García's insistence that the material component of man is "incapable of thought," Martínez writes that

> he knows little, exceedingly little, about the physiology of the intellect, of cerebral anatomy and pathology; the idea that the body is incapable not only of thought, but of feeling as well—what can he possibly know about mental illness? How the poor physiologist Magendie would laugh, he who established "that the brain is the material organ of thought." Poor poor Cabanis, unhappy Broussais, foolish Huarte . . . and all this, for what? To deduce a psychological truth—the immortality of the soul—from a physiological lie? Let's leave that half of the matter to theology and the Church.[101]

Continuing this line of attack, Martínez mocks García's naive dualism, inviting the author to produce "a speaking and thinking human soul separate from the brain," and ridicules the notion that the only thing capable of differentiating the matter in the mind of a genius such as Newton or Descartes from the matter in the simplest of plants is "this puzzle that is the *soul*, because without it there would be no self, and without a self there would be . . . a great mess of confusion and anarchy."[102] Martínez then advocates for an embodied self, challenging García to "study the brain with its connections and confluences and you will come to realize wherein resides the self of the general nervous system."[103] Ever sensitive to foreign perceptions of

Spain, Martínez closes by begging foreign experts not to pass judgment on his country's medical establishment based on a single text such as García's: "Foreign forensic scientists, physiologists, and anatomists, do not judge our understanding of mental pathology based on the book analyzed here. Heaven forbid that it has crossed the Pyrenees and that we must suffer the ridicule of certain cis-Pyrenean authors! No, no physiologists and distinguished physicians; mental pathology is more advanced among us than it may appear based on this book; please know that there are professors here who have much more solid knowledge of mental illnesses."[104]

In the subsequent edition of *El Crisol,* Martínez moved on from merely mocking Caballero to elaborating an argument that mental illness was a purely organic phenomenon and that an immaterial soul, whatever one's theological perspective, could have no influence. Martínez begins his article, "Mental Illnesses," by returning to the central question of whether "madness is a material or spiritual disorder, or to put it another way, are these illnesses organic or of the soul?"[105] He goes on to invoke his hero Juan Huarte de San Juan as one of the key writers on the topic, along with modern theorists such as Johannes Peter Müller, Johann Peter Frank, Broussais, and Cabanis. Martínez credits these various authors with sharing a common theory about the relationship between body and soul which can be summarized as follows: To the extent that souls are construed as spiritual entities, immaterial, identical, and immune to change, any and all variations in cognitive function, whether within the individual psyche or between individuals displaying different talents and aptitudes, must be the result of disparities in the physical organs through which the soul operates. Or, to put it in the words of Müller, "The activity of the soul depends on the integrity of the anatomical structure and chemical composition of the brain."[106] This state of affairs renders it impossible to attribute mental illness to a moral failing or spiritual deficit, according to Müller: "The physician should occupy himself only with aberrations in the intellectual faculties, only with material changes that incline the soul toward morbidity or impede its functioning; as a result, in the case of such organic alterations, we cannot assume an innate illness of the soul, as this would be a fundamental breach of the principle of morality, but rather a sudden change in the state of the brain instantly sickens the manifestations of the soul."[107]

Martínez sees an analogous doctrine in the work of Huarte, who wrote that the soul is greatly influenced by the body in the same way that a painter working with a high-quality brush paints better than a painter working with inferior tools. Moving on to the work of Johann Frank, Martínez quotes Frank's assertion that "manias are a type of illness no different from other disorders of the brain."[108] According to Martínez, Cabanis was correct in his insistence that "all man's faculties adhere in the brain; they are born, grow, change, increase, decrease, and are destroyed along with this material instrument."[109] Summing up, Martínez throws in his lot with the organicists, as a way of, counterintuitively, safeguarding the status of the soul: "In conclusion, we believe with Frank, Huarte, Broussais, Cabanis and the majority of authors, that madness is a material, nervous disorder and has nothing to do with any essential modification of the soul, because to introduce illness of a spiritual principle that is identical in all individuals seems to us absurd, immoral, and irreligious."[110] Interestingly, in this instance Martínez seems more receptive to the extreme localization of brain functions than he was in his earlier annotations on the works of Huarte and Sabuco. Here, he expresses confidence that, even though not all mental disorders have been linked to specific lesions in the brain, "we believe, with the organicists, that . . . in time these illnesses will be associated with organic characteristics, as has been the case with apoplexy, paralysis, and epilepsy."[111]

The Mind-Body Politic

Debates on the matter of mind were medico-political by nature, involving questions bearing on everything from jurisprudence to education to democratic self-governance. These debates were, in essence, attempts to offer competing diagnoses of social ills based on the interlocutors' preferred physiological, theological, and political frameworks. And like their early modern predecessors, they often availed themselves of the "body politic" metaphor in the process.

Félix García Caballero, for example, ends his treatise in precisely this way, describing the social cooperation necessary for maintaining the body politic: "Thus will man fulfill his mission on this earth: to be for society; and if society imposes on its members reciprocal duties in the interest of the common good, so too does it offer security and guarantees against the pretensions and abuses of its strongest members, establishing in this way peace and harmony between nations and the well-being of each and every member that makes up a given body politic."[112] García's body politic was predicated, however, on a collection of individual bodies separated from mind by an unbridgeable chasm: "Man, the most admirable being of creation, is a composite of two distinct substances: *soul* and *body*. Each of these elements of his being has essential attributes and properties—some dependent, others independent—that are subject to different laws appropriate to their different existences: the body, to the laws affixed by the Creator to matter; the soul, to those given to spirits by the Sovereign Maker, from whom they emanate and to whom they will return."[113] And this dualism, which Garcia saw as crucial to maintaining his vision of the body politic, was threatened by what he perceived to be the materialism of the organicist models of cognition championed by Martínez, and in particular the influence of phrenology, which had to be defeated according to García in order to forestall "the terrible and debilitating fatalism of the determinism to which the materialists condemn humanity."[114]

It is tempting to conceive of metaphor as superfluous to the real work of thought, a poetical oversimplification of more abstract concepts. But as George Lakoff and Mark Johnson have long argued, human cognition is grounded, via metaphors, in embodied experience, rather than situated in some rarified metaphysical realm.[115] From this perspective, the metaphor of the body politic is not a quaint rhetorical flourish, or a mere ornamentation of legitimate political theory; it must be seen, rather, as integral to the way humans conceptualize social relationships. Lakoff and Johnson's approach has been criticized, however, as ahistorical, lacking an appreciation for the context in which metaphors operate, and how this context changes over time.[116] For example, conceptions of medicine and politics changed dramatically in the span between sixteenth-century body politic metaphors and their nineteenth-century counterparts. The discovery in the seventeenth century of the circulation of the blood and the mapping of the lymphatic system, for example, presented new metaphorical source domains. Perhaps most strikingly, in the dissections of the brain undertaken by Gall, and the corresponding advances in the understanding of the nervous system during the nineteenth century, we can see the degree to which the body changed as a source domain over time. Similarly, political developments such as the challenges to absolute monarchy during the Age of Revolutions and the emergence of democratic mass politics over the course of the nineteenth century represent parallel transformations in the target domain.[117]

The body politic metaphor was ubiquitous in early modern Spanish medico-political literature, and the hierarchical emphasis of the metaphor was shifted in a meritocratic direction in the work of physician Jerónimo Merola and others. While analogies between medicine and politics often tended toward supporting the traditional status quo—in the work of conservatives such as Manuel Freyre de Castrillón, for example—nineteenth-century liberal physicians set about remapping medico-political metaphors, enlisting novel scientific disciplines such as physiology. Ildefonso Martínez, for example, availed himself of the body politic metaphor in his *Tratado de la fisiología*. In the treatise, he compares ignorance of the laws of society, which resulted in the dissolution of ancient societies such as Egypt, Babylon, and Carthage, to an ignorance of the laws of physiology, which inevitably results in the dissolution of the human body.[118]

One of the most striking examples of how these conceptual mappings evolved can be found in the pages of *El Porvenir Médico*, a medical periodical in which Ildefonso Martínez frequently published. In this case, it was one of Martínez's peers, the Catalán physician and progressive political activist Juan Amich, who penned several articles invoking a series of body politic metaphors that capture well the adaptation of the rhetorical device to the medico-political environment of mid-nineteenth-century Spain.[119] In September of 1853, Amich published a defense of Gall's doctrines in which he took aim at those who rejected phrenology "out of pride, without having studied it," and those, like Félix Garcia Caballero, "who believe it to be immoral and anti-religious."[120] In the article, Amich admits to being skeptical of Gall's work at first, but then becoming, after careful examination, a "partisan of his doctrine."[121] Much like Martínez, Amich attempts to reconcile an organicist model of cerebral localization with Christian theology and defend it against charges of materialism. In doing so, he holds that "the brain is divided into different parts, or organs, dedicated to particular functions,"[122] while at the same time insisting that the soul nevertheless remains free and indivisible; in order to exercise this freedom, however, the soul must avail itself of the brain in order to convey its directives to the rest of the body. In a body politic metaphor compatible with Spain's existing constitutional monarchy, Amich writes: "the soul is the sovereign of the understanding, and seated on its throne it convokes the organs which function jointly in order to communicate, when necessary, to the other organs so that they may obey the orders of the legislative power."[123]

By the following year the political situation had changed dramatically, and with it Amich's rhetoric. The July Revolution of 1854 brought to an end the moderate decade; it began with a series of spontaneous popular uprisings and resulted in the ascension of a progressive coalition which sought to dramatically democratize Spanish society. On September 15, 1854, Amich authored another article in *El Porvenir Médico* in which he deployed a revised set of metaphors. The article, "Politics and Medicine," begins by asking why most physicians tend to align themselves with democratic politics. Of course, there were many moderado physicians who did not, but Amich's characterization was undoubtedly accurate when it came to the readers of *El Porvenir*, a decidedly left-leaning publication. The answer was, according to Amich, that as men of science physicians are confronted by "laws dictated by nature rather than human intelligence," and what these laws demonstrate is a harmony of forces at work in the human body.[124] This harmony serves as the basis for a series of metaphors relating physiological processes to political systems. Interestingly, whereas before Amich had portrayed the soul as a sovereign ruling from its throne, he now insists on an organic equilibrium that equates to a vision of popular sovereignty:

> There is no organ which in its functions can be deemed sovereign; sovereignty resides in the whole, not in the parts; every system of organs is ruled by specific laws, and our economy can thus be compared to a number of confederated nations that offer each other reciprocal aid, and this harmony results in happiness and a social order that mirrors the health and life of the body. From the very moment in which a certain organ presumes itself superior, this excess results in illness, in the weakening of the other systems of organs, just as in the case of one or more nations dominating the rest, the result will be slavery; but the nature of man ensures a complete revolution in which either the whole triumphs as one, or dies at the hands of the part; there is unity because there is no interstice nor tissue which fails to energetically reject the diseased part; the body may succumb, but no one can deny the glory of its having taken the tyrant down with it.[125]

Amich then expands the body politic metaphor into a mind-body politic metaphor, in order to include the workings of the brain, which he conceives of as a self-organizing system composed of autonomous, independent neural circuits, each exercising its function in the service of the whole, in a manner he compares to a federal constitution that enshrines liberal political freedoms:

> Look carefully through the microscope at a nerve fiber, which in the midst of the encephalitic mass effects the marvelous phenomena of intelligence. Given these phenomena, what can we deduce from studying them? The impossibility of restricting their absolute liberty, because the Author of nature has decreed that they should exercise it completely. In this very same encephalitic mass we find a federal constitution, with each circuit working in complete independence and the others acting as mere auxiliaries; when a judgment is formed, memory, comparison, causality, circumspection, etc . . . serve as auxiliaries; if, instead, there is a desire to perform an act of benevolence or goodness, the active circuit, if it wishes, may consult with its counterparts and come to a resolution in total freedom. This is why we proclaim freedom of thought and conscience, freedoms which, like all others, cannot be limited.[126]

Amich's emphasis on freedom and equality entailed a program of social reform, which he goes on to outline; he decries "the wealth and pride of magnates juxtaposed with shacks in which hunger reigns" and bemoans the injustice that there "should be such a great distance between those who live in opulence and those who live in misery."[127] He then proceeds to employ yet another body politic metaphor, which in comparing the physical economy of the body with the financial economy of the state, argues for a more equitable distribution of resources: "In the normal state of our economy we have the experience of all our organs exercising their respective functions while simultaneously absorbing the nutrients they need. Why are not all social classes similarly protected so they can satisfy their needs?"[128]

Amich concludes his article with a defense of physicians' engagement in politics and a tribute to the medical profession as a vanguard of liberal political principles. He rejects the assertion that, because they were often employed by the government, physicians should be barred from political activism; a public post cannot deprive someone of their rights as a citizen, according to Amich. In fact, he continues, physicians are by the very nature of their duties predisposed toward liberal principles because these duties are based on "tolerance, amiability, [and] philanthropy," and are performed with equal care in response to the sufferings "of the absolutist as well as the republican, of the Catholic, the Protestant, or the Mahometan, each of whom may go wherever they please, and to whichever heaven they choose."[129] As was so often the case, this medico-political vocation was compared to a religious calling: "Physicians, as we are now like the priests in the early days of Christianity and the Middle Ages, spread throughout the land and interacting with all classes of society, it falls to us to exercise this exalted ministry so that all men are made aware of their rights and responsibilities; let us provide health to the sick, liberty to the people, and let us encourage philanthropy among the wealthy, then on our foreheads will rest the well-deserved laurels bestowed by God-made-flesh on Earth."[130]

On September 25, Amich published another installment of his series on medicine and politics, this time subtitled "A Study Comparing the Powers of the State and the Administrative Order with the Organization of Man."[131] Once again, Amich presented an extended body politic metaphor that drew heavily on the emerging scientific understanding of the brain. Amich's article addressed the fraught issue of the administrative apparatus, which in Spain, as elsewhere, was becoming ever more powerful as the government undertook ambitious infrastructure projects, intervened in the economy, and formulated increasingly detailed regulations in order to meet the complex demands of a modern, industrialized state. The growth of bureaucracy created inevitable opportunities for clientage and corruption, which could reduce a democracy to an oligarchy, or even a dictatorship, if "the elected leader were able to have the interests and destiny of the country at his disposal."[132] Amich sought to forestall this outcome through a study of the human body, summoning his readers to "discuss this important point and see if in the organization of man we find laws that may instruct us."[133]

In his analysis, Amich identifies analogues within the human body for the executive, legislative, and administrative powers of the state. The human body is portrayed as a "confederation" subject to the legislation of the physical laws of nature. Man is not a cause, but rather an effect of these natural laws, which can be seen as a legislative power outside ourselves, imbuing us with our functions and capacities. While the legislative power, this "great congress of the universe," is located outside man, the executive power resides within him in the form of intelligence generated by the brain. Here Amich resorts to a metaphor that had become increasingly popular since the 1830s, which likened the nervous system to a telegraph. This metaphorical construct was applied not only to the body, but often to the body politic as well, envisioning the telegraph as the nervous system of the nation.[134] Amich describes the human body as a system that functions by means of "the nerve fibers, which, like a veritable human telegraph, bring the various bodily functions into harmony with the intelligence, which we consider to be the executive power."[135]

The administrative order is, for Amich, subordinate to the legislative power, and corresponds metaphorically to the digestive and circulatory systems whereby the necessary nutrients are distributed to the human body just as the administrative state is responsible for distributing government services to the people. Summarizing his argument up to this point, Amich writes:

> The legislative power belongs to nature, and its constitution comprises all the elements, including man himself. The executive power, situated in the superior part of our being, is the intelligence, with the neural pathways putting it in relation to itself and to the exterior. The administrative order is divided between two great functionaries: the digestive tract with its lymphatic vessels that carry the liquids destined for the nutrition of the body, and the central circulatory system. It is this center that receives the sanction of the legislative power and is responsible for discharging it via the arteries, and thereby assimilating it throughout the entire economy. What we have here, then, are limitations on executive power, and the administration subject to the power of the legislature.[136]

Having laid out his metaphorical analysis, Amich proceeds to apply it to the contemporary political situation. Here he once again emphasizes the need for popular sovereignty, meaning "a number of individuals elected by the people and for the people, with the power to legislate, organize the administration, and name public functionaries, including the executive power." It is only through popular oversight of the executive power that "the harmony, health, and life of the people" can be assured, and a lack of such oversight will inevitably lead to the "sickness and death of the nation."[137] Constant vigilance must be exercised in order to avoid the depredations of excessive executive power, and here Amich deploys yet another body politic metaphor, although this time taking as his source domain a nonhuman body: "We must declaw the lion so that we will no longer be afraid. The claws of executive power consist in the ability to avail itself of the public goods of the country in an almost absolute fashion, thus giving rise to a rabid thirst for riches that will bring about the misery of the people, and once these riches are secured, they will be used to generously reward those in the employ of the executive, so that they become faithful servants of their master."[138]

The only bulwark against this state of affairs in Amich's view is the appointment of autonomous public functionaries who cannot be dismissed for partisan reasons. But what if, despite these safeguards, a public functionary becomes a creature of the executive power? In a final corporeal metaphor, Amich warns that such a creature must immediately be excised from the body politic before his "sickness contaminates his fellow functionaries."[139]

Political cultures, like most forms of culture, rely heavily on metaphors, and metaphors—especially body politic metaphors—were crucial to the development of new liberal political cultures in Spain. Tracing these metaphorical innovations and the participation of physicians in their development can provide insight into the relationship between medicine and politics in the nineteenth century. It also demonstrates the endurance of the body politic metaphor. The conventional wisdom on the body politic metaphor has been that it was inherently conservative and hierarchical, and that it succumbed by the mid-seventeenth century to political theorists such as Thomas Hobbes, who argued that the state was an artificial creation rather than a biological or natural entity.[140] More recent scholarship has demonstrated, however, that the idea of the body politic was much more persistent than previously thought, and more adaptable to a variety of social circumstances and ideological valences. In the English case, for example, Peter Elmer has shown that, contrary to the traditional scholarly consensus, the organicist notion of the state endured beyond the English Civil War of the 1640s, and that far from representing an inherently conservative politics, the metaphor of the body politic "continued to exert a strong fascination and unifying influence on men and women from across the religious and political spectrum."[141] This was the case in Spain as well, where the body politic metaphor—or, increasingly, metaphors of the mind-body politic—proved to be remarkably adaptable, not only to rapidly changing political realities, but also to novel physiological theorizing concerning the interactions between matter and mind.

CHAPTER 4

Medical Martyrs

Ildefonso Martínez was an avid devotee of the history of medicine; among his collected papers can be found historical studies such as the "Biographical-Bibliographical Compendium of Physiology," which detailed the progress of medical theory and practice from the Middle Ages to the nineteenth century. Martínez seems to have taken to heart the advice proffered by the *Boletín del Instituto Médico Valenciano* in 1842:

> One of the principal tasks that should be undertaken by one who dedicates himself to a scientific discipline is to compare its various epochs and the progressive development of its propositions and truths so as to form a precise idea of its current state and the advances that have been made. Unfortunately for us, medicine, which is the science that most demands this special study in order to precisely comprehend its different revolutions and systems, is also that which most lacks the philosophical works that enable a physician to understand the principles underlying the history of his art.[1]

Martínez's historical exploits were in keeping with a burgeoning interest in Spain's medical history, epitomized by works such as Antonio Hernández Morejón's *Historia bibliográfica de la medicina española* (*Bibliographic History of Spanish Medicine*) and Anastasio Chinchilla's *Historia general de la medicina española* (*General History of Spanish Medicine*). These works were pioneering studies in Spanish medical history, whose authors displayed a marked historicism—a recognition of the sociocultural determinants of medical thought—

yet at the same time insisted on the contemporary relevance of their historiographical project and its importance to the renovation of Spanish medicine.[2] Ildefonso Martínez was intimately familiar with these works; he cited them frequently and even reviewed them in the medical press.[3]

While Hernández Morejón and Chinchilla considered themselves first and foremost historians of medicine, their works contained political elements as well. Hernández Morejón, born in 1773, witnessed the early years of the liberal revolution, serving as a military physician during the War of Independence, and then going on to hold a chair in clinical medicine at the prestigious College of San Carlos in Madrid. During his medical career, Hernández Morejón simultaneously engaged in his historical pursuits, serving as a mentor to Chinchilla, twenty-eight years his junior, who was also working on his own history of Spanish medicine. Chinchilla had also started his career as a military physician and then went on to hold a number of academic posts. Upon his death in 1836, Hernández Morejón had yet to publish his work, but through the labors of his son-in-law it saw the light beginning in 1842, the year after Chinchilla began to publish his *History of Spanish Medicine* in serial form.[4] Both works combined a liberal disdain for the old regime and its hinderance of scientific progress, and a sense of wounded national pride at the neglect on the part of foreign scholars of the achievements of Spanish medicine. This aggrieved patriotism translated into a distinct nationalist bent in both works—an Enlightenment cosmopolitan nationalism in the case of the older Hernández Morejón, and a more fervid, Romantic nationalism in the younger Chinchilla.[5]

It is no small irony that, in his review of Chinchilla's work, Ildefonso Martínez criticized the author's nationalism, writing that he allowed himself to be "carried away by his patriotic enthusiasms."[6] Martínez himself was an avid liberal nationalist, and his writings provide a case study of how medical discourse could contribute to the construction of a liberal political culture for the new Spanish nation. The quintessential example of this dynamic was Martínez's treatise *Médicos perseguidos por la Inquisición española* (*Physicians Persecuted by the Spanish Inquisition*), published by *El Crisol* in 1855.

* * *

Wounded Healers

The endeavors of medical historians such as Hernández Morejón and Chinchilla were paralleled by the first attempt to chronicle the exploits of the Spanish Inquisition using archival sources, undertaken by the liberal cleric Juan Antonio Llorente. Llorente collaborated with the French forces during their occupation of the Iberian peninsula and participated in the dismantling of the Inquisition, beginning in 1808, which provided him access to the records of its various tribunals and ultimately led to the publication in 1817–18 of his *Critical History of the Inquisition of Spain*. Llorente's flagrant liberalism earned him the obloquy of monarchists in Spain, and he was forced to seek refuge in France upon Fernando VII's return to the throne. His reputation preceded him, however, and he was ultimately expelled by the French authorities for what were perceived as subversive activities.[7]

Even after the suppression of the Spanish Inquisition during the brief reign of Joseph Bonaparte, the status of the Holy Office remained a political issue, as the partisans of Fernando VII championed its restoration (succeeding in 1814) and liberals its ultimate demise (succeeding provisionally in 1823, and definitively in 1834). While the Inquisition as an institution had been moribund for over a century, it was transformed into a potent symbol by liberal polemicists like Llorente, and its fate came to be seen as a referendum on the kind of nation Spain was ultimately to become.[8]

In his treatise on persecuted physicians in *El Crisol*, Ildefonso Martínez drew on the work of Hernández Morejón and Chinchilla, as well as that of Llorente, and in so doing managed to combine two powerful themes: physicians as paragons of scientific rationalism and advocates for political reform, and the Inquisition as the epitome of an oppressive, reactionary old regime that stifled free thought, political progress, and scientific advancement. He begins the work with a pledge to "analyze medically" the Holy Office in order that his readers may "learn the lessons of the past," motivated by a "hatred for the executioners and tyrants of thought."[9] He then sets out, first, to record the names of the victims, and second, to relate details from the most famous trials of physicians conducted by the Spanish Inquisition. Following this approach, Martínez summarizes the cases of celebrated doctors such as Francisco López de Villalobos, the court physician to both Fernando of Aragon and Carlos V, who came under inquisitorial scrutiny due to his Jewish origins, and Juan de Nicholás y Sacharles, who was forced to flee Spain on account of his Protestant sympathies.

One notable exception to the litany of inquisitional misdeeds cataloged by Martínez was the case of Miguel Servet, the Spanish physician and Renaissance humanist who was not tried by the Inquisition, but rather put to death in Calvin's Geneva for the crimes of denying the Holy Trinity and infant baptism. Doctrinal differences notwithstanding, Servet's martyrdom served for Martínez as yet another example of the tendency of religious authorities to abuse their power, to become "jealous of their prerogatives," unlike Jesus himself, whose "gentleness, humility, charity, and benevolence, have rarely been imitated by Roman Catholics or by the Reformers."[10] The case of Miguel Servet inspired what was perhaps Martínez's most impassioned defense of intellectual freedom in his entire treatise:

> It is by no means strange that the inquisitors, that the reformers, should sacrifice the man who thinks, who desires, who believes differently than they do, because this is the effect of every school, of every doctrine, of every ordained authority. It is only a fully constituted individual liberty, which is to say one grounded in the inviolability of the human conscience, that is capable of respecting each and every individual idea, however extravagant, however exaggerated, however contrary to what passes as common sense. From this it follows that the moment there arises a privileged order, a school, an authorized church, there arises persecution, moral coercion, the punishment of dissidents, of skeptics, of those who think differently from the official, legal, accepted status quo.[11]

As he moves toward the conclusion of the work, Martínez draws analogies to the science of man and heralds medical science as the antidote to the intolerance and fanaticism of the past. The physicians persecuted by the Spanish Inquisition were "illustrious and dignified" heroes because "they remained true to their science." Martínez then cites the French writer and socialist reformer Alphonse Esquiros, who held that "Of all the sciences there is no other that touches more closely on the solution to the principle of liberty than anatomy and physiology" and predicted that "the philosophy of the future will be a physiology perfected."[12] Martínez concludes with a paean to his medical martyrs in which he once again credits science with dispelling the superstition and obscurantism that he held responsible for their tragic fates: "Here's to you, O great physicians persecuted by the Inquisition: yes, here's to you, illustrious martyrs; some of you suffered imprisonment, some the San Benito, others the bonfire, but your colleagues in the sciences have freed countless victims from your oppressors, and have replaced the executioners with charitable brothers!"[13]

Martínez's fixation with martyrdom was very much in keeping with the progressive reconceptualizing of the Spanish nation. This new narrative stood in opposition to the myth of an eternal Spain derived from the Visigoths, the Catholic kings, and Habsburg monarchs; it identified the true Spain instead with those persecuted for their beliefs, wrongly convicted, or forced into exile. Of this ideological project, Jesús Torrecilla writes:

> Having rejected the official Spain, they came to identify with all those groups that had been victims of the authoritarianism and intolerance of their rulers. . . . Having been denied their Spanish identity by those who would monopolize it as if they were its only legitimate proprietors, they proposed, in turn, that the truly authentic Spain was constituted of precisely those groups that had been amputated from the common trunk for defending their beliefs: the persecuted, the exiles, those adjudicated in the name of a truth that was not their own. Moreover, in identifying with those groups, they projected onto them their own ideas, as if being victims of the same kind of intolerance created a sense of intellectual community among them.[14]

Martínez's adulation of Huarte fits within this framework as well. Take, for example, the piece Martínez wrote in praise of Huarte in the *Círculo Científico y Literario* (*The Scientific and Literary Circle*), a prominent journal of the medical press. There he portrayed Huarte as the quintessential progressive reformer, whose critiques of the existing social order brought him into conflict with the vested interests of his day. Because he wrote on "the qualities that a king should have, not to mention what characteristics are required of judges, priests, physicians, and all the social classes," and because he dedicated himself to "attacking entrenched prejudices, censuring abuses, and exploring a path no one had tread before him," Huarte was, in Martínez's estimation, unfairly targeted by those whose privileges he threatened. Martínez lamented that Huarte wrote during "an epoch in which inquisitorial power was in full force," and speculated that, if he had lived in more favorable times, his doctrines would not have raised an eyebrow.[15]

A great deal has been written on how creative uses of the past helped construct the "imagined communities" of nationalist lore, and when it comes to early modern physicians as victims of the old regime, the intellectual community that writers like Martínez perceived was indeed an imagined one.[16] As is inevitably the case, the historical reality was more complex than the ideologically tinged narratives provided by progressive scholars such as Ildefonso Martínez. As Diego Gracia Guillén points out in an article entitled "Judaism, Medicine, and the Inquisitorial Mind in Sixteenth-Century Spain," while there is no doubt that physicians were persecuted by the Inquisition, they also collaborated with the Holy Office in pursuit of their own interests. Inquisition tribunals employed staff physicians, and such positions were both lucrative and prestigious. Among the duties of these physicians were attendance during torture sessions and providing diagnoses of prisoners who were thought to be mentally ill. But more importantly, medical discourse played a role in the widespread efforts to impose the social control that accompanied the rise of the early modern state. As Gracia Guillén puts it, "Medicine was a victim of the Inquisition, but it was also, and . . . to a larger extent, allied with the inquisitorial authorities in the task of corporally and morally disciplining sixteenth-century Spanish society."[17]

In his analysis, Gracia Guillén implicates the early modern medico-political tradition, and in particular the work of Juan Huarte. According to Gracia Guillén, during the sixteenth century, "while the Inquisition was becoming 'medicalized,' medicine in its turn, was becoming aware of its enormous political potential and its power as a disciplinarian of human conduct."[18] As we have seen, this new awareness inspired a long list of sixteenth-century treatises purporting to derive political insight from the structure of the human body and the practice of medicine, to analyze "the influences of the moral sphere on the physical one."[19] These include Enrique Jorge Enríquez's *Portrait of the Perfect Physician*, Jerónimo Merola's *Original Republic Derived from the Human Body*, and Oliva Sabuco's *New Philosophy of Human Nature*. And the tradition carried over into the seventeenth century, which saw the publication of a number of similar works, including Rodrigo de Castro's *Medicus politicus* (*The Political Physician*, Hamburg, 1614) and Cosme Gil Negrete's *Conclusiones medico politicae* (*Medico-Political Conclusions*, Madrid, 1654). Many of these books refer to Huarte by name, and all of them follow the idea that moral and social behaviors are determined by physiological processes, and that the physician could therefore intervene in order to control these behaviors, and in so doing govern the microcosm of the human body—just as the prince governed the mesocosm of the republic, and God the macrocosm of the world.[20]

Oliva Sabuco, for example, uses precisely this sort of language in her *Nueva filosofía*, referring to the human body as "the small world" and using it as a touchstone for part 3 of the work, entitled "Coloquio de las cosas que mejoran este mundo y sus repúblicas" (Colloquium on the Things That Improve This World and Its Republics).[21] The physician, according to Sabuco, is the "minister of the great secrets that God—and His secondary cause, nature—have created," and he must exercise his profession "with equity and justice," thereby "eschewing all that is misguided and injurious and substituting what is correct and useful for his patients and for the republic."[22] One important way the physician can serve the republic is through an understanding of heredity. In a chapter on marriage, Sabuco decries the common tendency to base marriages on economic factors and to forget that "the principle of perfecting human nature, as we see every day, is that the faults of the parents are seen in the children."[23] In this emphasis on the hereditary nature of moral qualities, Sabuco's medico-political doctrines approximate Huarte's, as Martínez points out in a footnote in his edition of the *Nueva filosofía*.[24] Sabuco closes the chapter with a passage of which Huarte would have approved: "When we desire a good horse, we go in search of a fine stud. Should we not likewise examine the man who would become a father and grandfather, so that he has good children and descendants, able men, and not beasts?"[25]

The doctrine that the heritability of physiological traits determined moral and spiritual qualities is also evident in Enrique Jorge Enríquez's *Retrato*, a work that draws on Huarte explicitly.[26] In keeping with his immersion in the tradition of Greek medicine epitomized by Galen and Hippocrates, Enríquez holds that the moral qualities of a physician are determined by his physical appearance: "The physician who has a handsome face cannot but be capable and skilled and have other qualities that are necessary for the perfect physician, since it is a philosophical rule that the customs of the soul follow the temper and complexion of the body, as Galen has shown in his book."[27]

When it came to such physiological determinism, as with the physician, so too with the king. Enríquez warns against monarchs with badly organized humors, as their hearts will tend towards irascibility, which when joined with great power is a dangerous thing.[28] The familiar equation of physician and king is a recurrent theme with Enríquez; both enjoy "great power" and have "subjects." The physician is king of the "little world" (*pequeño mundo*) of the body just as the monarch is the ruler of the republic.[29]

A tragic corollary to the widespread belief that moral qualities were rooted in biology, and thus heritable, was the antisemitism that characterized early modern Spain. The transmission of Judaism via the blood became a standard trope in debates about the status of the Jews and figured prominently in the construction of a racial caste system. Take, for example, Archbishop Juan Martínez Siliceo, a figure instrumental in the promulgation of the purity-of-blood statutes, who compared Spain to a stable in which inferior breeds of horses must be culled from the herd.[30] Such was the perceived power of Jewish blood that by the second half of the sixteenth century inquisitors were convinced that Judaizing could be instigated by the mere fact of having a Jewish wet nurse.[31] The same "moral biologism" that led to this antisemitism also served to privilege the aristocratic lineage of noble families, and according to Gracia Guillén took Huarte as a source of inspiration.[32] "This moral biologism naturally led to racism, that is, to the differentiation between noble and ignoble families, good and bad families, only by their blood or name. In reality this doctrine, which has in Huarte its major exponent, served to differentiate families by their blood. This suited the monarchy and nobility perfectly, and they gladly took advantage of it. The theme of blood purity served not only to isolate the Jews and the Moriscos but also to sanctify the nobles and kings, the 'bluebloods.'"[33]

While Gracia Guillén has provided an important corrective to the Romantic narrative that portrayed physicians as selfless martyrs, his own analysis, ironically, displays a similar lack of nuance. In presenting Juan Huarte as the driving force behind an unremittingly disciplinary medico-political discourse that culminated in the antisemitism of the purity of blood statutes, Gracia Guillén overlooks Huarte's philosemitism and his critique of inherited privilege. Indeed, as Jon Arrizabalaga and Maria Laura Giordano remind us, Juan Huarte praised the Jews as uniquely suited to the practice of medicine and rejected the discriminatory practices of the medical faculties of the time in favor of a meritocratic vision that privileged innate talent over aristocratic lineage.[34] And as we saw in chapter 2, Jerónimo Merola shared this meritocratic vision, and his treatise can be read as potentially subversive to the hierarchical social structure of sixteenth-century Spain. Just as the nineteenth-century science of man was a protean discourse with contradictory valences that could be deployed in a variety of ways, so too was its early modern predecessor. Turning now to Ildefonso Martínez's engagement with nineteenth-century theories on race, we will be confronted with the complex legacy of Huarte and the medico-political tradition of which he was a part.

The Science of Man and Scientific Racism

In his edition of the *Examen,* Martínez composed a lengthy note discussing human origins and the question of racial typologies. Such discussions were ubiquitous in the first half of the nineteenth century, as colonialist incursions, especially into Africa, initiated debates surrounding the perceived superiority of European civilization. By the 1830s and 1840s, these debates had become increasingly medicalized, as proponents of the science of man sought to explain the physical and moral differences between the various races.[35] Central to these debates was the controversy between monogenists and polygenists—those who saw humanity as a single species descended from an original pair versus those who considered different races as separate species. Monogenism had been the more prevalent view, as it was more easily reconciled with Scripture, but by the middle of the nineteenth century the secularizing forces of industrial modernity had increasingly brought polygenism into scientific fashion.[36]

Spanish authors produced various treatises on the science of man written from a spiritualist perspective that supported the monogenist view. A particularly influential exemplar was José Varela de Montes's *Ensayo de antropología* (*Essay on Anthropology*), which set out to explore the "intimate relationship that exists between the physical and the intellectual" aspects of man and argued for the monogenist position.[37] In a note to Huarte's *Examen,* Martínez took aim at Varela's essay and the spiritualist eclecticism it represented.

Varela de Montes's essay was intended as a didactic work for nonspecialists, and younger readers in particular, and in the prologue he claimed that his intervention into the science of man was necessary due to the profusion of organicist frameworks that sought to naturalize the spiritual aspects of human morality and cognition:

> If it had not been for recent efforts to put forth [man's physical] organiza-
> tion as an explanation for morality and the understanding, I would have
> limited myself to the physiological aspects of man; but when I see and hear
> it asserted that everything is a product of the organism, I must confront
> these questions, either to accept or reject their physiological basis, or situate
> them in their true terrain. This is even more necessary and urgent given the
> publication and profusion among our youth of works that materialize man,
> and make of his duties an arbitrary institution."[38]

Varela de Montes went on to assert that his ideological opponents were leading Spanish youth astray by sowing "venomous seeds" that would crowd out
"healthy and innocent" growth.[39]

In particular, Varela de Montes took issue with attempts to divide the
races in terms of intellectual abilities; he insisted that "A comparison of the
intellectual faculties of the diverse races does not justify dividing the human genus into distinct families," and that such attempts at classification
"bring no benefit and inevitably induce error."[40] Instead, according to Varela
de Montes, the human genus should be considered "a great nation composed
of 934 million individuals."[41] Ildefonso Martínez, in contrast, emphasized the
close linkage of intelligence to physiology, bringing to bear the work of Huarte as a foil to those "modern authors who attempting to be eclectics confuse
and contradict themselves at every step."[42] When it came to the assertion
that all races possessed the same intellectual potential, Martínez demurred,
arguing that Varela was blinded by his religious commitments, and that,

> In saying that everyone has the same intellectual capabilities, Sr. Varela gen-
> eralizes too much. If we are speaking in terms of the animating principle,
> or the rational soul, then we are in agreement, but this does not negate
> the observation that there exist essential differences in terms of intelligence
> from one type or caste to another. As we have already proven in some of
> our other notes, the differences in faculties depend on the greater or lesser
> degree of perfection in the [physical] organization, and not in any manner

on the soul, a spiritual substance we take on faith, but which is irrelevant to a discussion of the variability of intellectual capabilities between races.[43]

Martínez summarized the polygenist and monogenist schools of thought, characterizing them as "two of the most difficult physiological problems to resolve," and describing the former as the idea that "the human genus comprises distinct branches with distinct characteristics," and the latter as the idea that "the human genus is one . . . , and the differences in organization that exist between the varieties are due to accidental circumstances, such as climate, history, and habit."[44] In taking up these issues, Martínez pledged to "analyze them with the requisite judgment in order to deduce what we can with reference to the ideas of our Huarte."[45]

In addition to Huarte's insistence on innate psychological predilections, he also argued that environmental factors could shape individual and group aptitudes. In chapter 15 of Martínez's edition of the *Examen* (chapter 12 in the original), Huarte undertakes an extended analysis of environmental factors and their influence on the development of intellectual capabilities, describing the effects of climate and diet on the Jews during their sojourn in Egypt and how these gave rise to their "*genio*" for the practice of medicine. Huarte's analysis was remarkably similar to the fixation on climate and geography exhibited by the nineteenth-century science of man; Cabanis himself dedicated the entire ninth memoir of *On the Relations between the Physical and Moral Aspects of Man* to the topic of "The Influence of the Climates on the Moral Habits." In both cases, the emphasis was on the power of external forces to shape psychological attributes. According to Cabanis, "Every latitude has its characteristic, every climate has its specific aspect. But the different beings that nature has placed in them or that it reproduces in them every day, not only are appropriate to the physical circumstances of each latitude and of each climate, but also have a common stamp and, so to speak, aspect."[46] Huarte makes a similar claim in the *Examen*, wherein he invokes Galen's doctrine approvingly, writing that "Galen wrote a book proving that the habits of the spirit follow the temperature of the body wherever it happens to be, and for this reason the heat, cold, humidity, and aridity of the region that men inhabit, and the diet they consume, and the waters they drink, and the air they breathe [makes] some fools and some wise."[47] To which Martínez added in a footnote, "This proves that Huarte preceded both Cabanis and Broussais in considering the influence of the physical man on the moral man."[48]

In the *Examen*, Huarte provides a case study of the influence of climate in which he credits the desert heat of Egypt with fostering the aptitude of the Jews for the practice of medicine. According to Huarte, exposure to high temperatures results in a roasting of the choleric humor within the brain, a process responsible for fortifying the imagination, which he considered to be the faculty crucial for success as a practicing physician. In addition, he identifies other factors responsible for stimulating the Jewish penchant for medicine, such as the "subtle and delicate" winds and waters of the desert environment, and perhaps most importantly, the "manna" which, according to the Old Testament account, was a gift from God and formed an important element of their diet.[49] Given this environmental explanation of Jewish medicine's rise, the next step was to account for its persistence. This was made possible by the powerful influence of environmental factors on human heredity. In a Lamarckian vein, Huarte insists that acquired characteristics can be passed down through the generations; he asserts that momentary accidents can have generational effects, citing the example of a man who suffered a great fright resulting in a pallor that he subsequently passed on to his descendants.[50] By the same token, skin tones darkened by the sun in one region could endure for millennia in another; Huarte recounts a story in which, when God liberated the twelve tribes of Israel from Egypt, he also brought twelve Ethiopian men and twelve Ethiopian women into Spain, but despite the intervening years they had not lost their ancestral pigmentation. This was also true of the Roma who had, according to Huarte, emigrated from Egypt to Spain centuries ago, but had yet to lose their dark complexion, or the cunning and guile of their forefathers.[51] These examples demonstrate for Huarte "the force of the human seed when it is imbued with a deeply rooted quality," and leads him to conclude that, "in the same way that blacks passed on their color through their seed to their descendants without being in Ethiopia, so too did the people of Israel pass on their sharp wits to their descendants without being in Egypt, or consuming manna, because being stupid or wise is an accidental trait of a human, just as is being white or black."[52]

Huarte was not, however, positing a strict biological determinism. In his discussion of the Israelites he stresses their heroism and fortitude in the face of their desert exile and credits God with rewarding their diligence with manna from heaven.[53] This was, then, not an argument for an immutable Jewish bloodline, but rather a story of merit being recognized and rewarded, and this reward being passed down through the generations.[54] Martínez shared Huarte's esteem for the Jews, but when it came to countering the spiritualist anthropology of Varela de Montes, he resorted to a reading of Huarte that emphasized the more deterministic elements of his thought, which fit with the scientific racism that was coming to the fore in nineteenth-century Europe.

Having rehearsed Huarte's argument for the origins of the superior aptitude of the Jews, Martínez proceeded to deploy it against Varela de Montes in an attempt to prove the inferior intelligence of non-European races. Huarte's emphasis on environmental influences on human intellectual capabilities did not translate for Martínez into a sanguine attitude about the possibilities for achieving parity among the races, and this was in keeping with a widespread tendency among writers on race during the period. Whereas Enlightenment-era theorists evinced a decided optimism concerning the possibilities for human improvement, regardless of race, nineteenth-century anthropology increasingly emphasized the intractability of racial differences.[55]

Varela de Montes resisted this environmental determinism, admitting the influence of climate while asserting that it "does not have the power that it is all too often believed to have."[56] For Varela it was necessary to minimize the effects of climate in order to sustain his belief in the essential unity of the human family, especially with regard to the intellectual potential of the different races. He argued that, although there were differences in performance between human groups, these were not dramatic and could be rectified through education, and concluded that, when "the intellectual faculties of the diverse races are compared, it does not support the idea that the human genus is comprised of distinct families."[57] In the final analysis, Varela's doctrines rested on the conviction that human intelligence derived from an immaterial source; he cited approvingly Georges Buffon's investigations into comparative anatomy which resulted in the conclusion that "matter alone, no matter how perfectly organized, could not produce thought, . . . unless animated by a superior principle."[58]

This was where Martínez parted company with Varela—which is logical, given his strict biologism in the realm of human intelligence. In doing so, he completely sidestepped the issue of monogenism vs. polygenism. Martínez saw the debate between monogenists and polygenists as irrelevant to the question of the racial determinants of intelligence, as in either case there existed dramatic differences in physical organization that Martínez held to be dispositive. Whether these differences were due to climate acting on a single human lineage, or the legacy of the creation of distinct races as separate species, there would inevitably be a strong biological determinism at work. In the former case, the power of the environment to produce racial groups would presumably also result in the production of corresponding psychological traits and abilities among the members of these groups.[59] In the latter case, the power of racial typologies would be paramount, but the climate would not lose its influence on individuals, although the tendency would always be to revert to type.[60] In describing these two scenarios in a note on the *Examen*, Martínez begins with the monogenist position: "In effect, either the differences between the races depend on climate, or not; in the first case, there is not the slightest doubt that differences in organization depend on climate, and in this case, since intelligence is the child of organization (we have already proven that all souls are equal; to believe otherwise is both impossible and impious) it is easy to see that as varies the organization, so varies the intelligence."[61] He then moves to the opposing position, which held that differences in intelligence "do not depend on climate or diet, but instead depend either on the primitive organic composition of the races, which Mr. Varela rejects, or on the soul, an immaterial principle of which we know nothing, and whose existence we can only assume, while refraining from speculating about its activities."[62]

Such a position struck Martínez as incoherent, "whatever Buffon may say to the contrary," and he rejected it out of hand, insisting that science should limit itself to what can be observed: "What is certain is that no one doubts the existence of their own body, and when it comes to attributing properties, it is easier to posit the soul as a property of the body than to posit the body as a property of something that cannot be demonstrated by science, that reason can scarcely comprehend, and that while it may be accepted as a matter of sentiment, its existence can never be proved."[63] In conclusion, Martínez claims to have "proved all that is necessary" and to have argued for his opinions "forthrightly and without fear," and credits Huarte for pioneering an explanation for the disparities in human intelligence that combined an emphasis on the innate, organic disposition with an acknowledgment of the important effects of environmental factors.[64] Of these two causes, however, Martínez insists that "the primary disposition is the organic, and the second the climate and everything else that surrounds man."[65] Such an account of intellectual capacity was bound to be controversial, but not because it was patently racist—which it certainly was—but rather because it was materialistic. While Varela held out the possibility of mitigating racial disparities, like the vast majority of his contemporaries he believed that there existed in the present day a racial hierarchy in which the "peoples of the Caucasus are considered to be the most beautiful humans on earth," and in which there existed an "immense distance between the Caucasian and the Negro."[66] Thus, when it came to anticipating critical responses to his position, Martínez was not concerned with charges of racism, but rather with charges of materialism, and he sought to preempt them by touting his scientific integrity and religious bona fides, and, predictably, by charging his potential critics with adhering to a "disguised spiritualism": "We do not believe that we will be branded as materialists by scrupulous persons, but if it should happen, let it be known henceforth that we are religious without hypocrisy, and that we defend our philosophical opinions with reason, with no concern apart from searching for the truth, which we ardently seek and desire to find; and we do not believe that the truth is to be found in a so-called eclecticism, which is actually nothing more than a disguised spiritualism."[67]

But while Varela's spiritualism may have involved its own racist assumptions, it did not have the eugenicist implications that were evident in the work of Huarte. These implications were not lost on Martínez, who compared Huarte's account of the heritability of personality traits in the Jews and Gypsies to contemporary physiologist Antoine Louis Dugés's ideas on selective breeding:

This is an idea that a modern author of great merit has reproduced in our own day to convey the constancy of instincts in the different species and families of animals; it is based on the premise that character traits can be transmitted through generation, not just physical traits but rather dispositions, even educability, to the effect that a docile and well trained horse will produce a docile and well trained offspring, or one with a great capacity for learning—and such is the case with other species. This serves as a basis for identifying a perfect exemplar of the species for breeding.[68]

Huarte himself advocated a positive eugenics in chapter 17 of the *Examen,* where he sought to set forth guidelines for parents in order that they may "engender intelligent children" and thereby provide "the republic with the greatest possible benefit."[69] Because, according to Huarte, intelligence derived from a delicate balance between environmental and heritable factors, there was no guarantee that it would be simply passed down from parent to child; in fact, Huarte notes, we see that sometimes from "intelligent parents are born children who are idiots, and from parents who are idiots are born intelligent children."[70] Given this state of affairs, Huarte recommends a variety of interventions, from eating plenty of salt, to abstaining from sex for several days before attempting to conceive so that the man's sperm has time to "cook and mature."[71] Martínez dismissed Huarte's prescriptions for the most part, complaining that "in this chapter Huarte does little more than rehearse all the errors of the ancient physiologists," but he did entertain the prospect that Huarte may have been right to encourage unions between men and women of contrasting physiological makeups, and that if such a policy were put into practice it would alleviate a number of common diseases and "result in an improvement of the human species."[72]

Martínez elaborated on these themes in an article entitled "El higienista" (The Hygienist), published in the *Boletín de Medicina Cirugía, y Farmacía.* Deploying the eugenics of Huarte negatively, Martínez advocated the prohibition of marriage between "certain individuals suffering from illnesses that pose a threat to society," claiming that such a policy would contribute to "the improvement of the human species."[73] This policy was proposed in the service of a totalizing vision of hygiene as the "science of sciences," which would extend its purview not only to the institution of marriage, but to prisons, factories, the military, political institutions, the professions, and commerce. According to Martínez, "nothing would escape its penetration and study."[74]

As was his wont, Martínez managed to deploy Huarte opportunistically; while he repeatedly highlighted Huarte's advocacy of selective breeding, he also took an opportunity in his commentary on chapter 17 of the *Examen* to emphasize Huarte's acknowledgement of the vagaries of inherited intellectual ability, using this as a strike against hereditary aristocracy: "Here is one of a thousand arguments against a hereditary nobility: just because there was a great man who formed a hierarchy, it does not follow that his successors will be equally great; it is natural that nobility should be acquired personally, that is to say, through great and laudable actions in the service of one's country, not through pieces of parchment, however old, which may be useful when they deal with family origins and heraldry, but are useless when the successors of a hero are lazy and unqualified."[75]

In mid-nineteenth-century Spain, the majority of physicians followed the lead of writers such as Varela de Montes who advanced a thoroughgoing spiritualism grounded in Catholic teachings that was seen as a bulwark against the secularizing forces of modernity and a buttress to conventional morality and the prevailing class structure. Materialism remained a minority position—and this extended to attempts to bridge the gap between spiritualism and materialism, such as Martínez's "enlightened eclecticism." Mario Sánchez Villa has suggested that while this state of affairs may have retarded the development of a modern healthcare system in Spain, it may have also forestalled the wholesale rise of eugenicist policies that took hold in countries such as the United States and Germany.[76] Be that as it may, the eugenics espoused by Martínez foreshadowed the regenerationist rhetoric that emerged in the late nineteenth century and gathered momentum in the wake of Spain's humiliating defeat in the Spanish-American War of 1898.[77] The defeat was an international disgrace, resulting in the loss of Spain's remaining colonies, and was widely construed as symptomatic of a decomposition of the body politic. The cause of this degeneration was widely consider to be the deterioration of the Spanish race, and thus racial improvement came to be seen as paramount for the regeneration of Spain.[78]

Jews in the Mirror

Just as Juan Huarte appropriated the history of the Jews in the service of his preferred narrative of a meritocratic social order, Martínez, in turn, used Jewish history to bolster his vision of the old regime as intolerant and retrograde. In this telling of *la historia patria*, the Jews performed double duty as both medical and religious martyrs. Martínez advanced this vision in an 1855 work

that appropriated a format typical of early modern medico-political literature: the mirror of the physician. Following in the footsteps of authors such
as Enrique Jorge Enríquez, Martínez's *Espejo del verdadero médico* (*Mirror of
the True Physician*) offered up a prescription for the ideal physician, but in this
case one specifically tailored to a nineteenth-century progressive sensibility.

Indicative of this is the fact that Martínez wrote the *Espejo* under a Jewish
pseudonym: "Rabbi Isaac Maimon Firdusi." The rabbi, tellingly, shares the
same initials as Martínez, and some of the same ideological tendencies as
well; he identifies himself as a cosmopolitan figure who advocates tolerance
of religious and political differences in the interest of the advancement of
science. Martínez's alter ego displays his ecumenical tendencies in claiming
that his work directly incorporates the ideas of an unnamed Christian author, writing that, "although I am a rabbi, I am tolerant—so much so that the
second book of this work is a direct translation of a Catholic author, whose
views on the role of religion in the life of a physician I could not trouble myself to alter."[79] The rabbi also recommends the study of Arabic, as a familiar-
ity with the language will serve to "unearth ancient monuments of glorious
civilizations"—and in addition, the study of French, because it is the lingua
franca of European nations due to the status of Paris as "the Athens of modern times."[80] Like Martínez, Firdusi was an advocate of the science of man,
exhorting his readers to dedicate themselves "exclusively and conscientiously
to the study of man in his physical, intellectual, and moral aspects," and he
shared Martínez's fascination with martyrdom, insisting that aspiring physicians should "live as martyrs so as to die virtuously."[81]

Martínez's adoption of a Jewish persona was in keeping with an increasingly common tendency among Spanish liberals to idealize Jews as the quintessential victims of the old regime.[82] Works by liberal historians such as Antonio Puigblanch and Antonio Llorente cast the Inquisition's persecution
of the Jews as Spain's original sin, the initial dose of intolerance that ultimately came to poison the Church and the monarchy. As Michael Friedman
comments in his study of nineteenth- and early twentieth-century historical
treatments of Jewish Spain, "these widely publicized works brought renewed
attention to Spanish Jews and their descendants the conversos as iconic victims of a political system that a sector of Spanish Liberalism sought to over-
turn."[83] Puigblanch, like Martínez, demonstrated his identification with the
victims of the Inquisition by writing his critique of the Holy Office, *La In-*

quisición sin máscara (*The Inquisition Unmasked*), under the Hebrew pseudonym "Natanael Jomtob."[84] Such identifications were in keeping with the
tendency of Spanish liberals to dispute the master narrative of a centralized,
religious and ethnically pure Spain, and to substitute in its stead an emphasis
on a medieval coexistence, or *convivencia,* which reflected Jewish contributions to Spanish culture and sought to integrate the Jews into a revised version of Spanish identity.[85]

While at first glance it may seem strange that Martínez managed to unite
eugenics with philosemitism, this was not an uncommon combination for
Spanish liberalism. In fact, the racial improvement that was widely called
for in Spain came to be construed by many liberals as necessitating the re-
patriation of the descendants of the Jews who fled Spain in 1492. One of the
most notable proponents of this initiative was Ángel Pulido y Fernández, a
liberal Spanish senator. In Pulido's estimation, the medieval *convivencia* had
improved the Spanish race, and the expulsion of the Jews had been a "bloody
amputation" which had caused a "long and painful hemorrhage" in the body
politic.[86] Martínez's Firdusi reflects these sentiments as he declares a deep
affiliation with Spain: "Jew that I am, when I speak of Spanish authors I refer to them as 'ours' because I am directly descended from the Maimones de
Lara family of Spain, and although as a Jew I wander without a homeland, I
will always take Spain as my own."[87]

In Martínez's *Mirror,* the Jews were not merely portrayed as victims due to
their religious beliefs; they were cast as medical martyrs as well, having been
driven from the medical profession out of spite. Whereas Huarte de San
Juan had lauded the superior aptitude of the Jews for the practice of medicine, subsequent authors construed the prominence of Jewish physicians as
evidence of a devious plot through which the Jews had insinuated themselves
into positions of power and influence in order to undermine both Christian
morality and Spanish medicine. Typical of this type of polemic was the work
of Francisco Suárez de Ribera, which Martínez/Firdusi singled out for its
antisemitism.[88] In an early eighteenth-century treatise, Suárez lamented the
decline of Spanish medicine, which he attributed to the infiltration of crypto-
Jewish doctors into the profession. The practice of medicine, he complained,
"has declined due to some of its practitioners, namely, the Jews; these enemies
of ours, take up this profession in order to offend against Christ and against
Christians."[89] According to Suárez, despite the efforts of the Inquisition to

limit the practice of medicine to those of longstanding Christian lineage, doctors with Jewish blood remained, and thus he proposed the imposition of strict purity of blood requirements in the licensing of physicians: "Without a doubt, the Jewish physicians would be totally destroyed if the Holy Office were to require that whoever seeks to practice medicine or surgery etc. must present the required documents before the Holy Tribunal of the Inquisition, and that these, having been verified, would be passed along to the Royal Medical Board."[90]

Rabbi Firdusi replies directly to Suárez's calumnies; he pledges to "step forward in defense of my brothers, the Jewish physicians," whom Suárez had characterized as "duplicitous, arrogant, sycophants."[91] Firdusi turns the table on contemporary Christian physicians, charging that in fact "it is the Christian physicians of today who display these very same vices" and goes on in the second book to elaborate upon the familiar metaphor of medicine as a priesthood, but in this case one based on an ethic of universal religious tolerance.[92] In response to the "Catholic author" of book two, who insists that medicine should be grounded solely in "authentic and orthodox Catholic doctrine," Firdusi adopts the contrary position in a footnote wherein he writes that "the religion of the physician is humanity, the universal religion that takes man as the object of its study and meditations. He must be nothing less than tolerant toward all, and by the same token, whatever religion a physician may profess, he should fulfill his duty, if he indeed knows what it means to be religious—that is to say, human, and charitable in every sense of the word; *in omnibus charitas,* to quote St. Augustine."[93] This "universal religion," like the Catholic one, demanded self-sacrifice to the point of martyrdom in pursuit of one's spiritual ends, as Firdusi emphasizes in his description of the responsibilities of physicians during outbreaks of epidemic disease: "Any physician who fails to assist plague victims at the risk of his own life shall be considered outside the church, excommunicated, even if he does not receive a salary or any recompense whatsoever, for this is the greatest and most sublime act of his worthy ministry, and whoever fails in this should not call himself a physician."[94]

Martínez's idealization of Judaism was part and parcel of a distinct tendency among Spanish liberals—and especially progressives—to discern in the historical record reflections of their present-day preoccupations. Liberal intellectuals rejected the ideal of Imperial Spain in favor of what they perceived to be the democratic pluralism of medieval Al-Andalus, the resistance to political centralization on the part of the Castilian Comuneros, and the defense of the ancient *fueros* of Aragon.[95] This process of projection and reflection succeeded in creating a sense of community among progressives such as Martínez, but this community was a selective one; while in the abstract it aspired to a vision of universality, in reality it did not extend to women, for example, or members of non-European races. The medico-political tradition—both in its nineteenth-century incarnation as the science of man, and in its early modern manifestations, such as in the work of Huarte—was similarly ambiguous. It was not simply a discourse of social discipline and racism as described by Diego Gracia-Guillén, but neither was it a univocally liberal, modernizing force. The forms both these discourses took depended on the angles from which they were reflected in the mirror of contemporary political and cultural concerns.

CHAPTER 5

Spain in the
Time of Cholera

To this point, our investigation of medical politics in liberal Spain has focused largely on the role of medicine in the construction of new political cultures, cultures built of elements such as ideologies, discourses, and metaphors. But clearly medicine and politics are not merely questions of meaning—they are quite literally matters of life and death, as was tragically evident in the final years of Ildefonso Martínez y Fernández's life, which took place in the midst of violent political upheaval and pandemic disease. The revolution of 1854 and the virulent outbreak of cholera that accompanied it resulted in many casualties, Martínez among them, and generated heated debates in the medical press concerning the rights and responsibilities of physicians in both the political and the medical arenas. This period was also an eventful one in the medical press itself, with the advent of several new publications: 1853 saw the launch of *El Porvenir Médico;* in 1854 *El Siglo Médico* published its first issue; and in 1855 Ildefonso Martínez inaugurated his own journalistic endeavor, *El Crisol.* Given the diversity of their political orientations, these three publications offer a useful range of perspectives. Yet amid these differing perspectives appeared a shared disillusionment due to stalled reforms in the medical profession, a revolution that had gone too far, or not far enough, and the depredations of a cholera epidemic that had strewn chaos in its wake.

* * *

The Difficulties of Reform

At the outset of what would be the final year of Ildefonso Martínez's life, the medical press was in a retrospective mood, given the tumultuous nature of the previous year, which had witnessed not only a revolution and a deadly outbreak of cholera, but also a series of ambitious attempts to reform the medical profession. In January of 1855, *El Siglo Médico* looked back over 1854, which it referred to as an "eventful year, rich in promise and hope, but also in bitter disappointments."[1] Expectations were high at the beginning of 1854, according to the authors, given the prospect of a reorganization of the medical profession and the seemingly imminent approval by the cortes of a new law governing public instruction that had been designed by a commission of experts. In addition, a comprehensive sanitary law including quarantine restrictions that would encompass ports and adjacent hospitals for lepers, as well as other measures in the interior, was heralded as "conducive to the conservation of public health."[2] The article went on to present an extensive catalog of pending reforms such as a proposal to improve medical assistance to villages and the needy, an initiative to support the activities of the medical academies, and a project aimed at improving medical education. Given these ambitious plans, the editors had envisioned a "golden future" for these and other reform efforts that had long lain dormant.

The optimism that existed at the beginning of 1854, however, had not been borne out. "But all this has gone up in smoke!" lamented the editors. The blame was laid on the "tenacious resistance" that critics had deployed against these reform efforts, and the political chaos unleashed during the revolutionary summer of 1854. In addition, the brutal cholera epidemic that broke loose during the year played a role, which the editors acknowledged in a tribute to their colleagues on the front lines: "It merits special mention here the service of our colleagues who have fought a glorious yet ill-fated battle against the destructive monster that escaped from the muddy banks of the Ganges."[3] But according to the editors, the efforts of the government to meet the challenge of the epidemic did not measure up to the herculean efforts of the frontline healthcare workers: "What heroism on their part, what abnegation, what bravery and selflessness! But what carelessness, what humiliating disdain on the part of the government!"[4]

Reforming the medical profession was a project that had taken on an increasing urgency with the consolidation of the new liberal order, especially during the moderate decade, but given that the divisions among Spanish physicians were no less acrimonious than those within Spanish liberalism itself, this would prove to be no easy task. While many different reform efforts foundered in the face of the political and epidemiological realities of the revolutionary biennial of 1854–55, the problem was not merely situational; there are also patterns to be found in the welter of reforms that were proposed during the middle third of the nineteenth century. For example, physicians aligned with the moderado faction typically favored a course that centralized authority and decision-making in the hands of a limited elite of prominent physicians, much to the chagrin of their progresista counterparts.[5] We can perceive this pattern in the long-standing project of reforming the *partidos médicos,* or local healthcare districts. The partidos médicos were organized by neighborhood associations at the village level. Each district took responsibility for authorizing and facilitating the provision of medical services, but because there was little standardization or oversight in this process, the results could be arbitrary and capricious.[6] Wages were woefully insufficient; doctors were often paid in kind, and sometimes not at all. Consequently, the plight of rural physicians became a rallying point for the medical community throughout the nineteenth century.

A Central Committee for the Reform of Local Healthcare Districts (*Comité central para el arreglo de partidos*) had sprung up at the grassroots level and took on the ambitious task of overhauling the partidos, only to be usurped by a small group of well-connected physicians who were collaborating with the government's Council on Health, much to the dismay of the rank and file. Chief among these disgruntled outsiders was none other than Ildefonso Martínez y Fernández, who had been serving on the original committee. Martínez penned a letter to the editors of *El Siglo,* to which they responded in the paper's very first issue. With his typical lack of diplomacy, Martínez complained bitterly that those now in charge of the reform of the partidos were acting in bad faith, sitting on their hands, basking in their special roles without feeling any urgency when it came to providing actual results:

> As the reform of the districts has long been dormant in the government ministry, what power, what influence, what fate is responsible for the fact that it has not yet seen the light of day? Who knows? But we are persuaded

that if the aforementioned parties wanted, it would already be done, and those whom I represent would already be benefiting from the generous influence of their benefactors. This much is clear: it is not due to any impotence on the part of the physicians themselves that the reform lies sleeping and without direction, but rather to the apathy and inaction of these scientific luminaries.[7]

The editors responded to Martínez under an exceedingly thin veneer of professional courtesy, referring to him as the "learned and diligent physician D. Ildefonso Martínez," before going on to address his concerns in a response dripping with sarcasm: "It is an arduous task to discern the intentions of a writer; but if one were unaware of the healthy desires and loyal conduct of the author of this epistle, one could perhaps not be blamed for believing that the paragraphs transcribed here had the double motive of seeking popular acclaim while at the same time, with an elegance and grace capable of capturing the hardest of hearts, managing to shift the blame onto others."[8] They went on to accuse Martínez of positioning himself to take credit if the project succeeded, and evade responsibility if it failed: "If things turn out well. . . . Well, then we will have done it ourselves: the poor little *arreglo de partidos* was drowning, and we had the benevolence to pluck it out of the muddy and sandy waters of the ocean. In contrast, if things go wrong. . . . In that case, it's the fault of *the aforementioned parties,* the *luminaries,* just so we understand one another; it is that they are *impotent* (ouch!), *apathetic,* or *out of commission.*"[9] Ultimately, the editors of *El Siglo* were unapologetic about the exclusive and centralized nature of the endeavor.

Their vision was one in which the select few exercised their influence without the need to consult the *hoi polloi:* "It's true that various notable and influential physicians have intervened, and are intervening every day, using their good offices to insure that the project is published as soon as possible and presented to a prestigious consultative body."[10] And they went on to celebrate that this could be done without "the need for committees" and the "risky and ungodly agitation" they involve.[11] It seems that the editors' predictions of were borne out, as the report was indeed published later that spring. It appeared on April 5, 1854, with a preface by Prime Minister Luis José Sartorious.[12] But Ildefonso Martínez claimed to have been vindicated in the end.

The reforms were not a success, according to him; they were unpopular in the villages, and among the rural physicians who served them, since none of these constituencies had been included in the deliberations, and they were definitively derailed when the Sartorious regime fell during the revolution that broke out in July of that year: "You undertook a reform of the districts that involved a great deal of work, but because it was directed by the government without input from the medical classes, it was considered anathema in the villages and destroyed by the uproar of a political revolution."[13] For Martínez, this was a welcome defeat for what he dubbed the "medical aristocracy," a group whose members felt they deserved to be awarded "the cardinal's hat for their sermons to the government on improving the status of the medical profession."[14]

A similar dynamic was at work during the attempts to institute a centralized structure of medical colleges in Spain, to be presided over by a main *Colegio Médico* in the capital, similar to the Royal College of Medicine that had existed under Carlos IV.[15] Once again, it was an initiative that pitted a cadre of insiders with connections at the court against the corporative interests of those at the periphery. The effort was spearheaded by denizens of *El Siglo Médico* such as Mariano Delgrás and Francisco Méndez Alvaro—not to mention Martínez's sparring partner, Félix García Caballero.[16] At the inaugural banquet for the newly formed paper, held on New Year's Day, 1854, Méndez Alvaro described the initiative thusly: "The idea of establishing a Medical College in Madrid is an elevated and dignified one, which we should realize at all costs. This College, which we may refer to as Central, would oversee the other Medical Colleges which will arise in its shadow in the capitals of the various provinces, and they in turn will oversee the physicians in the rural areas, thereby creating a complete medical organization. Let us begin at the center. Let us toast to the creation of a Medical College in the capital of Spain."[17] While the project had the support of the government and seemed to be forging ahead, like the arreglo de partidos, the new plan foundered with the rise of a new governing coalition led by the Progressive Party in the summer of 1854. The political mood had shifted, at least temporarily, against the centralizing tendencies of the Moderate Party and toward the democratic aspirations of the popular classes—a shift that soon resulted in skirmishes in the streets of Madrid, and in the medical press as well.

The Revolution of 1854

The life of Ildefonso Martínez y Fernández was bracketed by two "paren-thetical" events.[18] He was born during the Liberal Triennial of 1820–23 and died during the Progressive Biennial of 1854–55. These episodes have often been dismissed as the products of failed revolutions, and themselves nothing more than ephemeral experiments in democratic politics, but in recent years historians have begun to reassess them, pointing out the global significance of the Liberal Triennial and the important role of the "crowd" in the Revolution of 1854.[19]

The Revolution of 1854 has been called the "forgotten revolution," coming as it did on the heels of the revolutions of 1848, with their pan-European character. And among Spanish historians themselves, the Revolution of 1854 has been neglected compared to other revolutionary events, such as the up-rising against the French in 1808, or the Revolution of 1868. But as María Zozaya has emphasized, other historians have seen the Revolution of 1854 as key to a better understanding of the role of popular protest in Spanish poli-tics in the nineteenth century.[20] While this neglected period warrants further analysis, my purpose here is not to reinterpret the revolution, but rather to focus on the medico-political response to it, both in the work of Ildefonso Martínez and in the medical press.

The revolution of 1854 brought to an end the moderate decade, during which the Moderate Party had governed in defense of oligarchy and in a fashion replete with corruption. The stage was set for the revolution by a con-fluence of factors including drought, famine, infectious disease, economic and governmental crises—but the ministry of Luis José Sartorius brought matters to a head. Sartorius, the leader of the "Polish faction," or *polacos*, named in ref-erence to his Polish origins, had made a precipitous climb to political power, as a journalist, having founded the periodical el *Heraldo* (the *Herald*), as a successful businessman, and as a deputy in the Congress in 1853, whereupon he was able to consolidate power as the leader of the cabinet. His power base inhabited the exclusive men's club, the Prince's Casino (*Casino del Príncipe*), which was peopled by the beneficiaries of the moderate decade, politicians and businessmen who had profited through the rampant financial speculation that characterized the Isabelline era in general, and the railroad boom in particular.

The backlash against the Sartorius government originated in the revulsion with the corruption occasioned by the feverish railway-construction boom, which lined the pockets of government officials. Critics on the progressive left denounced this corruption, considering it a betrayal of true liberalism, and calling for the overthrow of the government. But the crisis was set off in earnest by the Railway Draft Bill, which seemed to epitomize the government's malfeasance and caused even the allies of Sartorius in the Moderate Party to turn against him, and members of the military as well. The debate over the Railroad Bill became so contentious that the Senate was ultimately shut down and opposition papers closed. During this interlude, Sartorious took aim at military leaders he judged to be conspiring against him, posting them to remote locations far from the center of political power. This maneuver, however, merely succeeded in alienating the military and creating an even more determined opposition to the regime led by Leopoldo O'Donnell, Francisco Serrano, Facundo Infante, and others. And the dissatisfaction with the government was not merely among the military; radical groups on the left such as the *doctrinarios* were equally outraged. On February 20, a group of disgruntled military officers led an insurrection in Saragossa, but it was easily put down, initiating a wave of repression against the political opposition. After several months of playing cat and mouse, on June 28, O'Donnell officially declared himself in open revolt against the Sartorious government.

The revolution got off to a shaky start. O'Donnell received tepid support from the military, and the progressive wing of the liberal establishment saw little to suggest that their ideas would be taken into account. O'Donnell attempted to march on the capital but was turned away by government troops mustered by Sartorious at Vicálvaro. *La Vicalvarada,* as it came to be known, was not initially successful, but it set the stage for a wider uprising. O'Donnell retired to the south where he joined forces with the progressive general Serrano. On July 7, they issued the Manifesto of Manzanares, which laid out promises for reform and concessions to the left, which was enough to mobilize support throughout the country. Popular revolts sprang up among textile workers in Barcelona and rapidly spread to other cities across the peninsula. Ten days after the manifesto was issued, Sartorious saw the writing on the wall and stepped down, at which point Isabel ordered the formation of a new government.

The new ministry, led by General Fernando Fernández de Córdoba, managed to please no one and soon was faced with insurrection in the streets of the capital. The uprising began on July 17 at the bullfighting arena in Madrid, where a large group of laborers gathered in protest and requested that the musicians play the "Hymn to Riego," which had emerged as a revolutionary standard.[21] They were then inspired to march toward the center of the capital, and by midnight the city was in flames; barricades had been hastily erected in the streets surrounding the Puerta del Sol, and the residences of the queen and her various ministers were being vandalized. What had started off as a moderate coup attempt led by conservative military figures had become a popular revolution. For several days, the streets of Madrid remained barricaded while government troops attempted to restore order, shedding copious amounts of blood in the process. By July 19, Fernández de Córdoba and his associates Joaquín de la Gándara and Juan de Lara had mounted a sustained assault against the popular militias. As a participant recounted, "all of Madrid was a battlefield: there was blood flowing everywhere, everywhere echoed the volleys of gunfire, everywhere the roar of cannons. The hospitals were receiving the wounded nonstop, and were full of the blood of the troops and civilians alike; it was not uncommon to see an abandoned corpse, sometimes of a soldier and sometimes of a civilian."[22] Despite the best efforts of the military, the barricades were multiplying and the revolutionaries in the streets were able to hold off the troops. When it became clear that government forces could not control the uprising, the queen dismissed Fernández de Córdoba and called upon Espartero, who had remained sidelined up to this point, to form a new government led by the Progressive Party, thus bringing to a close the moderate decade.

The modest gains of the revolution did not last, however. As Charles Esdaile has explained, the Revolution of 1854 ended up strengthening the status quo. The revolutionary coalition was unstable in and of itself, and this combined with economic crisis and pandemic disease made failure a foregone conclusion. The leaders of the revolution, O'Donnell, Serrano, and Espartero, showed no interest in overthrowing the monarchy, or in heeding the bolder calls for radical social reform, and as a result, the popular revolution stalled.[23] In addition, the agenda of the Progressive Party was hampered by disorder in the countryside occasioned by food shortages resulting from excessive grain exports, and by the ravages of cholera.

The revolution was a radicalizing moment for progresistas like Martínez, some of whom were moved toward republicanism by the events of 1854. While Martínez was already quite radical during the moderate decade, his writings during the Liberal Biennial suggest that he, like many of his peers, was disillusioned and frustrated by the unfulfilled promises of the revolution. Evidence of this attitude can be found in an essay written in October of 1854, "Letter from a Deaf-Mute to General Espartero," in which Martínez's mouthpiece excoriated the vacillations of the Progressive Party, thus giving us a valuable indication of Martínez's own political commitments at this juncture.[24]

Because he cannot hear, the narrator of the essay declares himself impervious to the political speech that corrupts others: "I am, Your Excellence, deaf, and consequently I disregard rumors that I cannot hear, gossip that I cannot understand, and criticisms that are lodged in vain against me. Because I am deaf to all this, I will pursue my path with nobility and independence."[25] Likewise, because he cannot speak, the narrator claims to be incapable of "calumny, rhetorical tricks, or dishonorable utterances."[26] As a result of these impediments, the deaf-mute insists that only the purest of ideas have been able to penetrate his mind, and these have in turn produced infallible intuitions, the study of which have taught him "the worth of revolutions," and "what contributions are made by revolutionaries."[27]

This conceit provides Martínez the rhetorical framework for his observations on the political situation in the wake of the July Revolution. In a warning to Espartero, he remarks, "Yes, Your Excellency, you are surrounded by snares, caressed by enemies, resting on your laurels, smug and self-satisfied in your victory, but nevertheless, there is so much to do."[28] In a bitter denunciation of the timidity of the progresistas in the hour of their apparent triumph, Martínez insists that the enemies of liberty must be confronted: "There are so many to be taken care of, but we have taken a seat so quickly; there is so much that needs to be destroyed, and we have given up so soon; there is so much to be known, but we have learned nothing, even through our disgrace; there are masks to be ripped off, yet we allow everyone to dance away, obscured by the facade of liberty."[29] Martínez chastises those "who proclaim themselves liberals" but who since the July Revolution "want to profane the sacred tree of liberty, while basking in its shade."[30]

Martínez then makes a parallel to 1843, the year that a progressive coalition succumbed to the Moderate Party at the start of what would become the moderate decade, when General Narváez had forced Espartero from power. Invoking Espartero's ignominious fall, Martínez writes: "Attention liberals! Attention Espartero! The events of the year 43 should be a harsh lesson for you. Learn, once and for all, not to be weak nor generous with your enemies. . . . Would it were that we had a Washington! But contrary to the pretensions of many self-proclaimed 'great men,' the Spain of today is the land of Lilliput. We are nothing more than dwarfs. Dwarfs in our politics, dwarfs in literature, revolutionary dwarfs."[31] Martínez goes on to exhort his readers not to shrink from the demands of the hour, explaining, "These are not ordinary times. This is a revolutionary epoch, and revolutionary in the progressive sense, today more liberal than yesterday, and tomorrow more than today."[32] He then issues a warning against a sense of complacency that too often afflicted liberalism in his opinion, apologizing for his heated rhetoric, but claiming it to be necessary given the urgency of the situation: "I have learned through my solitude, through study, through experience, that tranquility, and tolerance, and the kiss of peace afforded to traitors only serves to embolden them and allows them to laugh at our expense, to ridicule us, to make fools of us, because there is no greater foolishness than to give our enemies the opportunity to make martyrs of us. This is liberal idiocy."[33]

What progresistas must do, according to Martínez, is to have the courage of their convictions and seize the moment. Referring once again to the "sacred tree of liberty," he writes: "It is the grave fault of the so-called progressives to fear a tree which yields such ripe fruit, and it is a grave error on the part of men such as Espartero to fear liberty, from which we can only expect benefits, and yet show no fear of despotism, which inevitably leads to the gallows."[34] For Martínez, Espartero's allegiance to Isabel II lay at the heart of the matter; if Espartero was determined to pay obeisance to the current dynasty, then the future was a "foregone conclusion." But if he were willing to make a radical departure, there was hope. Invoking the standard catalog of revolutionary martyrs, he urges Espartero to throw in his lot with the far left:

"No! And forever no!" exclaim from the grave the immortal Riego, the ill-fated Laci and the brave Porlier. "Learn, learn, and free yourself; do not be stubborn as we were, do not believe in flattering promises, because when you come to your senses it will be too late." . . . Zurbano clamors from the tomb, "I fought for the throne and the constitution. What did that throne make of me? What did that despotism make of me? A martyr. Open your eyes Esteemed Sir; do not fear liberty; do not crush it—Don't let them guide you! Don't let yourself be indoctrinated! What do you stand to lose with the ultra-liberals? Nothing, absolutely nothing! In fact, you stand to gain much more than you would by indulging in half measures."[35]

Martínez then asks, rhetorically, how the typical moderation of the liberals has benefited them: "you have been expatriated, kidnapped, left to rot in Logroño. In being cooperative, liberals have suffered every damage imaginable. You would have been better off carrying the revolution to its ultimate and logical conclusion."[36] Martínez continues, invoking his hero Riego as an example of what happens to liberals who lack the courage of their convictions:

> If Riego on July 4 had used his prestige to mobilize the people and execute that perjurer of a king, would he have suffered a worse fate than being executed himself? Certainly not! He was executed because he lacked the courage to be an executioner, to execute someone that he had every right to under the law—and he would have done so if he had been a true revolutionary, but he was not, and so he was hung after being dragged to the scaffold in a basket, he who had just three years earlier been paraded through the streets in triumph, in a cart pulled by generals.[37]

Martínez begs Espartero to shun Riego's example and to act decisively, because "despotism does not care if you are more or less liberal, only that you have been marked as an enemy."[38] The only remedy against the machinations of authoritarian rulers is, according to Martínez, an unwavering commitment to liberty, because "that is what tyrants and those partial to them hate."[39] Drawing another historical parallel with 1843, Martínez insists that Espartero's power is proportional to the degree of his support for the liberties of the people, and then as now, the danger is that his retinue will lead him astray, that he will again suffer the loss of faith of the *pueblo*. The antidote to such an outcome, insists Martínez, is the recognition that the monarchy and the aristocracy are the enemies, and that the lesson to be learned from 1843 is the futility of compromise: "If you had broken with the throne courageously and with revolutionary fervor, you would not have suffered exile, but you temporized, you accommodated, and the institution took advantage of your weakness, whereas it would have been defeated by a strong figure such as Cromwell or Napoleon."[40]

Seemingly unfazed by the contradictions involved in invoking Cromwell and Napoleon as unalloyed champions of democratic liberties, Martínez forges ahead in his outright advocacy of republicanism, casting the issue in terms of "the eternal struggle of the monarch against the people."[41] The central weakness, according to Martínez, is deference to the queen, and it is this deference that constitutes Espartero's fatal flaw. Martínez then begs Espartero to take a harder line against his enemies, given the nature of the forces arrayed against him:

> Hear me General Espartero, for once listen to the voice of reason: do not be so generous, do not put such faith in your own strength or the strength of your party, be suspicious of those who surround you, make war against apostasy, free us from the bloodsucking leeches of the state, cut their budgets and put yourself resolutely on the side of the taxpayers rather than the bureaucrats. Create a government that is thrifty and just, and you will merit our congratulations, and those of the whole nation. But if you are too trusting, as in the year '43, if you heed the bureaucrats and lack the courage to make radical reforms, . . . then your future, your prestige, will dissipate more and more each day, because actions speak louder than words. . . . If you think you can make your grandchildren the beneficiaries of your reforms, those living today will lose their patience and you will be held responsible by God and man. If you do nothing when you could have done everything, your historical legacy will be that of a weak man of little wisdom and less courage, and all your prestige, glory, and patriotism will be dismissed as vainglory.[42]

There is no sign that Martínez's diatribe was ever published, but as subsequent events would come to reveal, his concerns about Espartero's weaknesses were not misplaced.

While his appeal to Espartero may not have been made public, in another instance Martínez did make a very public display of his feelings toward the revolution. In November of 1854 Martínez delivered a speech on the thirty-first anniversary of the execution of Rafael Riego, in the plaza where he was executed, and in front of a makeshift shrine composed of portraits of the fallen hero, his military decorations, and the catafalque that bore his coffin at his funeral. In the speech, Martínez connected Riego's sacrifice with the Revolution of 1854, lauding the "victorious and heroic nation of July the 18, 19, and 20," and he urged his compatriots to contemplate the shrine in honor of Riego as "the apotheosis of a martyr for liberty," who was "one of the many victims of the tyranny of Fernando."[43] Continuing in this vein, Martínez decried the king's bad faith, exhorting his audience: "Behold, every one of you, this sad example of the fickleness of fate, the rancor of tyrants, the force of violence directed against free men. Behold, patriots, the reward given by kings to their faithful servants."[44] But it was the moderados, in Martínez's estimation, who had done the most damage to Riego's reputation, spreading damaging rumors accusing him of being a republican and an anarchist, and in so doing they had "done more damage than the royalists."[45]

Periodicals, Politics, and Pestilence

Just as the period 1854–55 was a turbulent one in the political sphere, there was a great deal of upheaval in the world of journalism as well. The year 1855 saw the creation of new medical periodicals, and given the state of the public sphere, and of public health, there was no shortage of controversy for the medical press to cover. *El Siglo Médico* was launched in 1854, and the advent of this new periodical stirred up controversy in the medical profession and the medical press, which was chronicled in the pages of *El Crisol. El Siglo Médico* was launched by bastions of the "medical aristocracy," Francisco Méndez Álvaro and Matías Nieto Serrano, via the merger of two prior publications, the *Gaceta Médica* and the *Boletín de Medicina, Cirugía y Farmacia*. As the merger was cheekily described in *El Crisol*, "in the month of January a new periodical appeared, the natural born child of the legitimate marriage of the old *Boletín* and the youthful *Gaceta*, and the child was christened *El Siglo Médico*." But no sooner had this child came of age than "the rowdy troublemaker began to pick fights with everyone, while at the same time carefully observing the etiquette appropriate to the official organ of the medical bureaucracy."[46] This characterization captures *El Siglo's* combination of pugnaciousness and moderate liberalism. An analysis of the disputes between *El Siglo* and *El Porvenir* during this period provides an interesting window on the confluence of medical politics with social reform and pandemic disease.

The fight picked by the "rowdy troublemaker" in the summer of 1854 began as a dispute over public health, but quickly took on political overtones. During this time, the world was bearing the brunt of the third great cholera pandemic (1846–60), which is thought to have originated in India and spread through Europe, Asia, Africa, and North America. The stage was set in Spain for a deadly outbreak of cholera in 1852 due to a subsistence crisis caused by a harvest that only delivered half of the accustomed amount. The famine intensified the following year, and by the fall of 1854 the disease had secured a beachhead among a malnourished populace in Galicia. In the edition of July 2, José Varela de Montes, one of the editors of *El Siglo*, lambasted physicians in Vigo, in the province of Galicia, for casting doubt on the outbreak of cholera there. In doing so, according to Varela, they had given support to "the errors of a credulous and ignorant populace."[47] Rather than keeping the controversy within the medical profession, however, Varela called upon the government to take legal action against the skeptical physicians, thereby bypassing the traditional immunity of physicians in such matters. This *trahison des médecins* was not taken lightly by other medical periodicals, and a searing broadside was soon forthcoming from the left-leaning *Porvenir Médico*, but not before the outbreak of the July Revolution, and as a result the ensuing back-and-forth became a strange combination of a debate over public health and an exercise in revolutionary rhetoric.

The criticism levied by *El Porvenir Médico* combined outrage for the perceived wrongs done to the physicians in Vigo with an ascription of political motives to *El Siglo*. The editorial in *El Porvenir* refers to *El Siglo Médico* as "*El Siglo polaco*" in reference to the polish origins of prime minister Luis Sartorious, who had presided over the corrupt and ineffectual government that had become the target of the July uprising. Tarring *El Siglo Médico* with the sobriquet "polaco" was a sharp rebuke on the part of the editors of *El Porvenir Médico*, associating, as it did, *El Siglo* with a reactionary and corrupt status quo.

The article begins with a denunciation of the "crime perpetrated by *El Siglo Médico*" against the immunity of the medical profession, and goes on to condemn "the Polish periodical" for indulging "the ruinous instincts of these reactionary figures."[48] The editors of *El Siglo* stood accused of betraying the most vulnerable members of the medical profession: the *médicos de partido,* those provincial physicians laboring in poverty and obscurity. According to *El Porvenir, El Siglo* had advocated the prosecution of the Vigo physicians for questioning the existence of cholera in the region, and in so doing had jeopardized "that most noble prerogative, the sacred immunity of the profession." In essence, *El Porvenir* was accusing *El Siglo* of making it a crime to deviate from accepted opinion—as defined by the editors of *El Siglo.* In closing, *El Porvenir* emphasized again the role of *El Siglo* as a tool of the establishment, characterizing its editors as "base adulators of power" and urging the physicians of Vigo to stand firm against the "shady machinations of the medical club" while vowing to throw their words in their face the next time the editors of *El Siglo Médico* held forth on their supposed commitment to the medical profession which they "denigrate, humiliate, and degrade."[49]

Although the editors of *El Porvenir Médico* sought to paint *El Siglo Médico* as a tool of the now defunct Sartorious regime, *El Siglo* was not unsympathetic to the July Revolution. In fact, the paper saw the revolution as a golden opportunity to advance the interests of the medical classes and repeatedly called upon physicians to avail themselves of the moment to achieve long-awaited reform by functioning as moral exemplars and by getting involved in electoral politics. In general, however, they proffered the image of the physician not as an agent of radical social change, but rather as a stabilizing influence in times of political unrest, such as the present moment. In their August 13 edition, for example, the editors of *El Siglo* did not engage in unmitigated celebration of the revolution, but rather assumed a more subdued tone, praising the medical profession for its level-headedness "on the battlefield" or in "civil disputes," wherein a man "takes up arms against his fellow citizens, his friends, and even his own family." In such circumstances, when the combatants are "blinded by fury and overcome by the sanctity of the cause they are defending, they only think of damage and destruction. And there, where the most terrible passions scarcely leave room for reflection, there, where hatred and vengeance reign, appears a man, serene and tranquil, full of charity, of love, of science, exposing himself unarmed to the deadly hail of lead in order to bring comfort to the defeated and placate the wrath of the victors. This man is the physician-surgeon."[50] And if this image of surgeon-saints minis-

tering to the wounded was perhaps too subtle, the editors went on to characterize medicine as an adjunct of the Christian faith, employing the familiar
analogy of the physician as priest: "Ah! Medicine is the second religion of
humanity and those who practice it are priests dedicated to the most sublime
virtue of the true religion."[51]

The editors of *El Siglo* placed physicians in line with the spiritual powers
that be, in hopes that the common people would come to fully appreciate the
medical profession and extend the requisite gratitude toward "those who rate
so highly in the realm of civilization and morality!"[52] According to the editors, states prosper when the medical classes "are well trained, honorable, and
zealous," and when they attain the corresponding societal benefits. But how
to engineer this rise in status and education so badly needed by the medical
profession? To answer this question, the editors refer to the reforms of the
clergy undertaken by the liberal regime in previous decades when salaries
had been regularized and dioceses were redrawn more rationally:[53] "Do we
not see how the government provides special protection to the ecclesiastical
estate, arranging affairs so that the number of clergy is adjusted according
to need, and thereby assuring that each will enjoy the decorous subsistence
required for them to adequately fulfill their exalted mission?"[54] The editors
went on to draw a similar parallel with public education: "Do we not see the
government intervening, as it should, on behalf of primary education, determining the qualifications that teachers must have, authorizing them to teach,
and setting their salaries?"[55] Without such protections, the editors argued,
"it will be very difficult for the medical profession to serve society as it can
and should." And this assistance was only fair, they continued, as physicians
bore the brunt of caring for the sick, "without defense against the very same
pestilences, without rest, and without a moment of leisure."[56]

The editorial tenor of *El Porvenir Médico* was quite different from that of
El Siglo; it was characterized by a more celebratory tone with regard to the
July Revolution, and adopted a much harsher rhetoric toward the governing
elites. In the immediate aftermath of the uprising in Madrid, for example, *El
Porvenir* published an animated editorial singing the praises of the revolution:

We would be remiss in our duties if we failed to address, however briefly,
the glorious political revolution that we are experiencing, a revolution that

will occupy a distinguished place in the annals of history, and one that will place Spain at the level of the most civilized and cultured of nations. . . . The present revolution has no party; it is a national uprising in which the honor and dignity of all Spaniards has risen up against the immorality and prevarications of the governing class; it is an idea that was once oppressed now breaking its chains; it is political liberty putting tyranny in its grave; it is right triumphing over might; and, at last, the restoration of the principle of the LAW, and of MORALITY.[57]

The editors' enthusiasm for the revolution is obvious. They claimed to be unable to contain their "joy at the hard-won objectives" of the uprising, and saw in it a bright future for the medical profession, and a rebirth of the "glories of la medicina patria." Despite the unifying rhetoric, however, to secure this rebirth a meticulous examination of the "medical corps" (*cuerpo médico*) would have to be undertaken: "In order to achieve this regeneration of the medical corps, as with the physical body, it is necessary to undertake a careful diagnosis, to scrupulously examine all the pathological elements which are causing pain, to measure carefully their strength and malignancy, to search for an appropriate remedy and apply it with discernment but without fear, with sound judgment, but also with courage."[58] The editors predicted that such an examination would unsettle the "medical club," since it would jeopardize their "scandalous acquisitions" under the previous, corrupt administration. For the partisans of *El Porvenir Médico*, *El Siglo Médico* was unmistakably part of this discredited medical club.

While *El Siglo* cast the physician as moral exemplar, *El Porvenir Médico* took the analogy one step further, exhorting the medical profession to supplant the clergy's traditional role among the common people, and to undertake a "sacred mission" that would involve actively evangelizing new ideologies in the public sphere: "this work, which must be undertaken today with unwavering ardor, is precisely to inculcate among the people the idea of liberty, to explain that which they do not understand, and to demonstrate the falsity of the preoccupations that have been malevolently nurtured among them."[59] It was up to physicians to provide this political education because they enjoyed the trust of the residents of the small villages that dotted the countryside of Spain, and, *El Porvenir* assured, they would receive the thanks and blessings of their charges as soon as they came to appreciate and understand the benefits of true liberty. And in addition to providing this "incalculable benefit to the country," the medical profession would see its social influence grow and physicians "would come to exercise a direct and powerful influence on the administration of the state." This was the only way, according to the editors, that "science will come to be appreciated in all its value, and the reforms that the medical profession demands may be solicited directly from the seats of parliament, and not in the antechambers of the offices of government ministers." Through these means, the editors proclaimed, "our patriotism and our professional enthusiasm will assure the triumph of liberty in Spain, and situate our beloved science in the elevated position that it should occupy."[60]

The more radical position staked out by *El Porvenir* was also possibly the result of generational dynamics; the editors highlighted generational fissures within the medical community, anticipating that while "a noble, loyal, and patriotic spirit has guided our pen," there would be those who took issue with their ideas, an old guard who would seek to maintain their entrenched positions of power. In response, the editors saw themselves as creating a "moral bulwark" against the "excessive ambition and sinister plans" of those who would block the rise of a new generation of physicians by availing themselves of "condemnable schemes," all in the service of "defending their salaries." Closing with a threat, the editors promised that, should such actions occur, they would "be more explicit and let the truth be known to the medical profession," calling out the perpetrators by name.[61]

Such assertiveness in the wake of the Revolution of 1854 would prove fleeting, however. In an indication of how fragile left-wing enthusiasm for the revolution would prove to be, on September 30, 1854, an article appeared in *El Porvenir Médico* decrying a recent government order prohibiting physicians from changing residence—presumably in order that they not flee impending outbreaks of cholera. The article decried the new, so-called "liberal and enlightened" government, and in so doing provides an indication of the difficulties faced by the new progressive regime and its inability to institute meaningful reform in the face of a raging pandemic. In response to this infringement upon the freedom of movement among physicians, the author writes: "*What kind of country are we living in?* . . . We have spoken with a great number of physicians, and they all ask the same question in astonishment: How is it possible that this comes from a liberal government, the product of the July Revolution, whose banner, stained by the blood of the people, displayed the precious words *liberty* and *morality?*"[62] The order was seen as an insult to the profession, whose members, as the author points out, had already been "willingly sacrificing themselves in order to save the lives of the sick . . . without the threat of ridiculous punishments."[63] The author suggests that if the government wants to treat doctors as public functionaries and to "punish them the moment they fail in their duties by abandoning their posts," then it should at least pay them a living wage. If not, then it should leave them alone.[64] Such was the disgust with the political direction of the new government that the author refused to even rate it above its predecessor, declaring that both were "bad and defective."[65]

Indeed, the new progressive regime found itself hamstrung from the outset, undermined not only by the advancing cholera pandemic, but also by food shortages brought on by a series of poor harvests, and by political upheavals occasioned by resurgent Carlists on the right and labor unrest on the left.[66] Faced with such fierce headwinds, the new government shied away from undertaking radical reforms: the queen was allowed to remain on the throne, and Espartero's new cabinet did not include so much as a token member of the Progressive Party.[67] Ultimately, the fears of Martínez's *sordo mudo* would prove prescient; Espartero could never bring himself to break with the monarchy and embrace the goals of the popular revolution, and by 1856 he had squandered his reputation as the "people's general" through his constant truckling to the forces of conservatism. Espartero's betrayal of the left, however, gained him no support on the right, and in July of that year he was forced to step down in the face of yet another uprising, led by military strongman Leopoldo O'Donnell, whose political inclinations were more in keeping with the *status quo ante* of the moderate decade.[68]

The frustration surrounding the issue of government control over the movements and ministrations of physicians during the cholera epidemic, reflected in the pages of *El Porvenir Médico,* would prove to be a continuous source of controversy in the final year of Ildefonso Martínez's life, during which he would return to his home province of Asturias in order to assume a new post, and where he would be drawn into a fateful conflict between his duties as a physician and his own self-preservation.

To Oviedo

In April 1855, Ildefonso Martínez assumed the position of director at the Fuensanta mineral baths in Buyeres de Nava, located thirty-five kilometers from Oviedo, the provincial capital of Asturias. Martínez's journey to Buyeres was a circuitous one; five years earlier, Martínez had applied for the very same post at Fuensanta but ran afoul of the Byzantine process through which medical posts were awarded in mid-nineteenth-century Spain.

During the period, positions were awarded according to scores made on public examinations, and on April 10, 1850, the *Gaceta Médica* announced the examination for positions at the mineral baths, and added that this news was "sure to attract attention now that such events have become so infrequent, to the great detriment of science and the medical profession."[69] According to the *Gaceta*, the judges appointed to assess the examinations were "known not only for their erudition, but also for their firm principles and their independence and impartiality."[70] Somehow, these qualities failed to secure Martínez's desired outcome. Despite achieving the highest score on the placement examination, he was not awarded the position.

Commenting on the situation, the editors of the *Boletín de Medicina, Cirugía, y Farmacia* wrote, "It is lamentable that Sr. Don Ildefonso Martínez, after finishing in first place for the baths at Buyeres de Nava, was not offered a position. . . . It is our hope that the government will realize his merit and find some way of using his excellent abilities."[71] The editors of the *Gaceta* weighed in on May 30, writing that, while a Dr. Mestre had been appointed director of the mineral baths at Buyeres de Nava,

> this choice has left the gifted young Dr. Ildefonso Martínez without a position, despite the fact that he was the top-scoring candidate for the mineral baths at Buyeres and has undergone many other examinations with equal success. The government must have had its reasons for preferring Mr. Mestre, but we see no reason for denying Mr. Martínez the post that he earned via a public examination, and consequently the government is in some sense obligated, if it is to proceed logically and fairly, to rectify the harm that he has suffered, through no fault of his own, and secure for him another similar position without requiring a new examination.[72]

This campaign in the medical press seems to have borne fruit; a new position materialized by royal order on June 21, 1850, and shortly thereafter Martínez was listed in the *Gaceta Médica* as the director of the mineral baths at Bellús in the province of Valencia.[73]

Despite the skewed results of the examination, Martínez remained a believer in the importance of public placement exams for medical posts as a means of establishing a meritocracy within the profession. Writing five years later in *The Mirror of the Perfect Physician*, Martínez recognized the flaws in the system but insisted it was preferable to one based on clientage and imposed by the government: "That the examinations as conducted at present have serious defects has been well documented and is beyond doubt; but despite their flaws, they are preferable to direct appointment on the part of the government."[74] In his evaluation of the various critiques of the current system, Martínez even described the precise scenario he himself had encountered: "Another objection to the placement exams concerns one of the typical outrages perpetrated by the officials who organize them: naming the second- or third-place finisher the winner and leaving the first-place finisher without a post."[75] Continuing in this autobiographical mien, Martínez insists that the medical press must play a key role in ensuring the legitimacy of medical placement examinations, writing that, going forward, the "medical press, the scientific press, should take up in each issue any faults in the integrity of the process," and that in doing so journalists will provide independent perspectives and "will not put forth rash judgments, but rather function as faithful interpreters of public opinion."[76]

In the end, it seems that Ildefonso Martínez was able to navigate the system to his benefit, having negotiated an exchange of positions with the current director of the baths at Fuensanta in the spring of 1855.[77] But in achieving his long-sought professional goal, Martínez had put himself in the crosshairs of the global cholera pandemic that was beginning to manifest itself across northern Spain and would soon wreak havoc in Asturias.

As the disease spread, debates abounded concerning the proper measures to adopt in the face of the threat. One of the most contentious of these revolved around the issue of quarantine policy. The medical press was full of articles by liberal physicians on the need for stricter measures while businesses pushed back against these measures, denouncing them as an infringement of the fundamental liberal belief in free markets. As *El Siglo* pointed out in June of 1855, in Spain as elsewhere, commercial interests were exerting pressure to relax quarantine policies, and this was evidenced by the amendments to a bill in the cortes sponsored by one deputy Figuerola. After celebrating the election of "fourteen or sixteen professors of medical science" to the cortes, the editors lay into Figuerola as an "ardent defender of mercantile interests" who surprised the cortes with what amounted to a "complete annulment of our quarantine system."[78] In the interest of maintaining economic growth, Figuerola had proposed to weaken the quarantine protocol in Spain. *El Siglo* denounced this decision, decrying the fact that it would leave Spain "open henceforth to cholera," and predicting that, "as a result, thousands of Spaniards will pay with their lives in exchange for a negligible commercial advantage."[79]

Méndez Alvaro put it even more starkly in *El Siglo,* where he decried the "apathy" and "indifference" of all the nations of Europe:

> What do the nations of civilized Europe do when faced with a scourge that impoverishes and depopulates? Apathetic and indifferent, busy with their deadly wars and dominated by politics, which is the mania of this century, as every century has its mania, greedy for the quick and easy riches of the free market, and forgetful of the fact that man is the primary and principal element of wealth, as it is he who produces it with his mind and his arms, they undertake only the most basic hygienic measures, more often than not of doubtful efficacy.[80]

Méndez Alvaro goes on to lament the failure of European countries to coordinate their efforts, insisting that any solution must be a European-wide one in which the various governments across the continent come to an agreement on how best to "extinguish the pestilence at its source, to uproot it in the climate that gave rise to it and the causes that originated it." The only way to accomplish this, according to Monlau, was to establish an effective quarantine regimen throughout Europe. Absent these measures, the risk was that the disease would become endemic in Europe.[81]

El Crisol was equally insistent on the need for strict quarantine policies—one of its few areas of agreement with *El Siglo Médico. El Crisol* lambasted efforts to weaken quarantine restrictions and strongly declared a belief in the contagiousness of cholera, declaring that "we are contagionists, not by caprice, but by simple induction and practical experience. We have spent the last six months fighting cholera . . . and have followed its progress with interest and without fear, and although our limited scientific knowledge may have little value in the eyes of eminent men . . . maritime quarantines [and] closed borders all corroborate the contagionist position, and the latest wave of cholera from France brought many over to our side."[82]

This uncharacteristic agreement between *El Crisol* and *El Siglo* in their opposition to the lobbying of commercial interests highlights the medico-political significance of cholera, a significance that cut across the entire spectrum of nineteenth-century European liberalism. Cholera represented an insult to liberal notions of progress and a challenge to the competence of the emerging liberal state. It amounted to a double bind in which efforts to safeguard the liberal order threatened to undermine widely espoused liberal values, such as the free circulation of ideas and goods, property and capital.[83] In the end, cholera would have the last word; despite the expressions of indignation among liberal physicians, the disease continued its tragic itinerary.

As discussed previously, in the early days of the epidemic some physicians denied they were dealing with cholera—they insisted that it was instead an outbreak of typhoid—but by the fall of 1854 cholera was indisputably on the march, and deaths were officially being recorded as due to "cholera of a bilious nature." It was clear from the outset that the disease was preying especially upon those whose health had been compromised by famine, the poorer classes both in the rural areas and in towns and cities. On November 6, the Civil Register of Oviedo recorded a death in the parish of San Julián de los Prados as "suspected cholera," and from that point cases spread like wildfire, leaving 273 dead by the end of December.[84] Despite these losses, January of 1855 was rung in with great optimism that the scourge had run its course.

This optimism was tragically misplaced, however, and by the summer of 1855 cholera had returned to Asturias, prompting the City Council of Oviedo to convene an emergency meeting on August 30, 1855.[85] The council lamented that the previous year's outbreak had severely depleted the city budget and proposed a levy to cover the costs of fighting the disease. On September 1, the council met again to reimpose the public health measures that had been in force during the previous outbreak, assigning physicians to direct relief activities in each of the six districts of the city.[86]

Ildefonso Martínez, having recently taken up his position at the nearby mineral baths, was ordered by the governor of the province to come to Oviedo on September 5 in order to treat victims of the cholera outbreak.[87] It is not clear why the governor insisted on Martínez's presence since he was already fully engaged with the epidemic in Buyeres, where he had authored a treatise on the disease and was immersed in the treatment of cholera victims.[88] In fact, this may have accounted for his failure to present himself to the authorities in Oviedo as scheduled. Two days after the initial summons, Martínez had yet to appear, and it was only on the evening of September 9 that he finally arrived in the capital.[89] On September 20, the municipal government determined that the outbreak was on the wane and freed Martínez from his duties.[90] However, for reasons unknown, Martínez remained at his post, and on September 26 he died of cholera at the age of thirty-four.[91]

At the end of a literary career filled with allusions to martyrdom, Ildefonso Martínez can be said to have died a martyr's death. The precise circumstances surrounding Martínez's demise, however, remain shrouded in mystery. While some sources characterize his journey to Oviedo as purely voluntary,[92] his official summons by the governor seems to have been controversial even among the editors of *El Siglo Médico*, who in a tribute to Martínez harshly criticized the action taken by the governor, characterizing it as "violent" and "capricious," and declaring that, if "we lived in a country that was competently governed, the Governor of Oviedo would not escape a bitter punishment for his conduct."[93] Continuing, the editors expressed their dismay at the passing of Martínez, despite the ill feelings that had come between them: "La medicina patria has lost a passionate enthusiast, noted for his erudition and extensive expertise. It gives us great pain to have lost a person for whom we have always had great esteem, despite the fact that our friendship was not what it once was."[94]

Pedro González Quiros Isla, in an article on Martínez, speculates that political calculations may have been behind both the initial failure of Martínez to secure his desired post and what he considers to be the governor's unjustified summons of Martínez to Oviedo.[95] González cites the contrast between Martínez's progressive political convictions and the conservative tenor of the moderate decade as a possible reason for the decision to deny him the directorship at Fuensanta in 1850. Regarding the governor's decision five years later, he cites the fact that there were eight other physicians in the capital at the time, a number he deems adequate for dealing with the epidemic, and points out that there was no shortage of cholera victims in Buyeres de Nava in need of Martínez's care. This suggests to González that the governor bore some sort of animus against Martínez. While these scenarios are plausible, there is no way to judge definitively the motives behind the decision to call Martínez to Oviedo.

One further piece of evidence adduced by González can be dismissed, however. Curiously, in support of his theory that government officials bore ill will toward Martínez, he claims there was no tribute to him in the records of the City Council of Oviedo, when in fact the council paid homage to Martínez in an extended entry in the Municipal Record on the day of his death.[96] On the evening of September 26, the mayor lamented the passing of Martínez:

> Today I have the bitter task of announcing the tragic death of the able and honorable physician D. Ildefonso Martínez, director of the baths at Fuensanta, which occurred at 3:00 this morning, the result of a sudden and fatal attack of cholera. The City Council has an urgent duty to fulfill today—to consecrate a monument in memory of the accomplished and distinguished professor Martínez in order to perpetuate his virtues, his abnegation, and the zealous perseverance with which he dedicated himself to the care and treatment of a wretched and suffering humanity.[97]

The council agreed to provide a perpetual resting place for Martínez's remains in the local cemetery, with a marble plaque to be inscribed with a message that "transmits to posterity the name of this erudite and distinguished physician who fell victim to his honorable and charitable zeal to assist the sick."

Conclusion

Having come to the end of Ildefonso Martínez's life, the inevitable questions arise: What does his life ultimately signify within the broader context of the liberal revolution? How can we definitively situate his work with regard to the major currents of intellectual activity in mid-nineteenth-century Spain? In sum, what does he represent? Unfortunately, there is no easy answer to this question; in fact, I tend to agree with Hans Renders that it is not a particularly useful question to begin with: "Too often a biography offers an incentive for historians to declare a person's life story to be representative of a grand historical narrative. However, to expand our knowledge of the past, it is more useful to test whether a grand narrative needs to be corrected and made nuanced precisely because of the interpretation of the life at hand."[1] Like many idealistic young physicians of his generation, Ildefonso Martínez was passionately committed to the reform and regeneration of the medical profession. Indeed, he took this commitment to extraordinary lengths in his engagement with professional associations and in his journalistic exploits. And like so many of his peers, Martínez was immersed in the project of creating a new political culture for liberal Spain; his historical scholarship was part and parcel of this process, and true to form he made significant contributions with his editorial interventions and commentaries on key works in the Spanish medico-political canon—and all of this condensed into a brief, fifteen-year span, beginning with his first public presentations in 1840 and ending with his death in 1855. With these facts in mind, we might say that he was very much a man of his time, only more so.

But simultaneously, the life and work of Ildefonso Martínez are difficult to pigeonhole. For every polarity that one may draw, Martínez defies expectations. His strident anticlericalism, for example, was paired with a sincere Christian faith that went well beyond a deracinated Enlightenment deism. Although we do not have any record of his explicit religious convictions, it is clear that he took great pains to show that his work would not undermine religion. While he was decidedly a left-wing progresista in his politics, this did not translate into a straightforward alignment with positivism and experimentalism, and a rejection of vitalism, as prior scholarship would predict. Likewise, his championing of heroes of early modern Spanish medicine, such as Oliva Sabuco and Juan Huarte, was on the one hand designed to advance the narrative of an ascendant scientific rationality being thwarted by religious authorities, while on the other to provide a bridge between science and religion, between materialism and spiritualism. And despite his vision of a medical vocation that went hand in hand with political advocacy directed toward "universal emancipation," egalitarianism, and democracy, his medico-political theorizing countenanced both sexism and racism. Thus, during his brief life, Ildefonso Martínez y Fernández managed to engage with a remarkable panoply of issues in the medical politics of mid-nineteenth-century Spain, but in ways that revealed various complexities and contradictions.

Perhaps Martínez is an example of the "exceptional normal," to use Edoardo Grendi's well-known formulation.[2] For Grendi, as for Renders, the issue is not representativeness but the additional historical insights that emerge from microhistorical analysis of obscure or neglected figures. The goal here is not to arrive at a fixed explanation of the relationship between the individual and the collective, as Sabina Loriga reminds us. Taking her cue from Wilhelm Dilthey's suspicion of "totalising concepts," Loriga writes, "An individual cannot explain a group, a community or an institution, and conversely a group, a community or an institution do not make it possible to explain an individual. There is always a disparity between these two poles, and this disparity is inexhaustible."[3] For Loriga, the "tension" and "ambiguity" generated by this disparity is not to be avoided, but rather celebrated and embraced.[4] Daniel Meister makes a similar point, arguing that historical biography should "chart a middle course" between these extremes, alternating "its gaze between the subject and their context."[5]

I do not wish to engage in methodological hair splitting or revisit the extensive theoretical debates concerning the relationship between biography and microhistory. In the final analysis, I concur with Meister's assertion that historical biography should move beyond these debates and that it "does not require its own theorizing."[6] The work of historical biographers, like that of other historians, emerges out of archival encounters, sometimes serendipitous, always messy, with source materials that promise to shed new light on the equally messy reality of humans and their societies. It is then a matter of bringing to bear whatever conceptual frameworks and theoretical approaches are deemed most appropriate. This kind of methodological bricolage has guided my analysis of Ildefonso Martínez y Fernández, and while individual cases cannot form the basis for wholesale revisions of historiographic frameworks, they can help bring to light the complexities of a historical period. The historiography of nineteenth-century Spain has often been prone to stark polarities and sweeping generalizations. It is my hope that this study can contribute to a renewed appreciation of the intricacies and subtleties of the era.

Notes

Preface

1. The inventory of Martínez's works was compiled by archivist Mercedes Cabello Martín in 2011. See "El Archivo Personal de Ildefonso Martínez y Fernández," 1815–45, BH AP 4, UCM Biblioteca Histórica Marqués de Valdecilla.

2. See, for example, "Medicinal Monarchy," in Keitt, *Inventing the Sacred*. My initial exploration into the life and work of Martínez was published as "Medical Martyrs: Nineteenth-Century Representations of Early Modern Inquisitorial Persecution of Spanish Physicians."

Introduction

1. Although this is the first comprehensive study of Ildefonso Martínez y Fernández, there have been some brief biographical sketches over the years. One of the earliest was written by Constantino Suárez Fernández in 1936, but its publication was delayed until 1956. See Constantino Suárez Fernández, *Escritores y artistas asturianos: indice bio-bibliográfico*. On Martínez's friendship with the celebrated essayist and bibliophile Bartolomé José Gallardo, see Gútiez, "Ildefonso Martínez, amigo y bibliotecario de Gallardo." Other useful biographical details can be found in González Quiros Isla, "El Dr. D. Ildefonso Martínez y Fernández. Una víctima del cumplimiento del deber." Delfín García Guerra and Víctor Álvarez Antuña provide an account of Martínez's contribution to the identification of pelagra in Spain in their book, *Lepra asturiensis*, 72–85. In an indication of more recent interest in Martínez, since I began the present work, some of Martínez's writings have been made available online ("Ildefonso Martínez Fernández 1821–1855," www.filosofia.org/ave/003/c018.htm).

2. The indispensable work on the science of man in France and its many permutations is Williams, *The Physical and the Moral*.

3. See, for example, Arquiola, "La incorporación a España de una visión utópica de la medicina," 105–19; Novella, "Medicina, antropología y orden moral en la España del siglo XIX"; Cepedello Boiso, "La influencia de Condillac y los ideólogos en la teoría del derecho española decimonónica," 148–56; and Sánchez Villa, *Entre materia y espíritu*. One of the few English-language works touching upon the science of man in Spain is Haidt, "Emotional Contagion in a Time of Cholera."

4. On this movement, see Siraisi, *History, Medicine, and the Traditions of Renaissance Learning*.

5. The secondary literature on Huarte and Sabuco is so vast that it is only possible to provide the briefest of overviews here. A classic work on Huarte is Iriarte, *El doctor Huarte de San Juan y su Examen de ingenios*. The most recent and comprehensively annotated edition of Huarte's *Examen* is Juan Huarte, *Examen de ingenios para las ciencias*, ed. Guillermo Serés. Serés examines the politcal aspects of Huarte's thought in "Huarte de San Juan: de la 'naturaleza' a la 'política.'" For a general treatment of Huarte in English, see Read, *Juan Huarte de San Juan*. There has been a tendency to view Huarte as a critic of supernaturalism and as a precursor of modern psychological and neurobiological theorizing. See, for example, Bustamante Martínez and Martín Araguz, "Examen de ingenios, de Juan Huarte de San Juan, y los albores de la neurobiología de la inteligencia en el Renacimiento español," and García García, "Huarte de San Juan, un adelantado a la teoría modular de la mente." For an exhaustive bibliography of works pertaining to Huarte, see Molina Cantero, *Juan Huarte de San Juan y su Examen de ingenios para las ciencias*.

In the case of Sabuco, general treatments include Torner, *Doña Oliva Sabuco de Nantes*, and Henares, *El bachiller Sabuco en la filosofía del Renacimiento español*. As in the case of Huarte, there have been many connections drawn between Sabuco's work and modern brain science, such as Guy, "Miguel Sabuco, psicólogo de las pasiones y precursor de la medicina psicosomática"; Martín Araguz, "Spanish Brain Science and Philosophy of Mind in the Time of Cervantes"; and Martín Araguz, Bustamente Martínez, and Fernández Armayor, "El suco nerveo sabuceano y los orígenes de la neuroquímica en el Renacimiento español." Unlike the case of Huarte's *Examen*, there have been several modern English translations of Sabuco's work. See Sabuco de Nantes y Barrera and Miguel Sabuco, *New Philosophy of Human Nature: Neither Known to nor Attained by the Great Ancient Philosophers*, ed. Waithe, Colomer Vintró, and Zorita, and Sabuco de Nantes y Barrera, *The True Medicine*, ed. and trans. Gianna Pomata. Other secondary sources of interest, in no particular order, include Balltondre Pla, "El conocimiento de sí y el gobierno de las pasiones in la obra de Sabuco"; Bidwell-Steiner, "Metabolisms of the Soul: The Physiology of Bernardino Telesio in Oliva Sabuco's Nueva Filosofía de La Naturaleza Del Hombre (1587)"; Plastina, "Oliva Sabuco de Nantes and Her Nueva Filosofia"; and Arroyo, "Giving Birth to Science: Oliva Sabuco and Her Intrusions into the Male Episteme."

The attentive reader may have noticed the switches between "Oliva" and "Miguel" as authors of the *Nueva filosofía*. This stems from a protracted dispute over the authorship of the work. In 1903 José Marco e Hidalgo discovered documentation that he claimed showed that it was in fact Oliva's father, Miguel Sabuco, who authored the book. This assertion has been strenuously contested by María C. Vintró and Mary Ellen Waithe in "¿Fue Oliva o fue Miguel? Reconsiderando el caso Sabuco"; in Waithe and Vintró, "Postumously Plagiarizing Oliva Sabuco: An Appeal to Catologuing Librarians"; and in the introduction to their translation of *La nueva filosofía* referenced above. Other scholars have pushed back against these defenses of Oliva Sabuco's authorship; see, for example, Pretel, "El enigma Sabuco: el parto de los montes." Because the dispute does not show signs of being resolved any time soon, and because the authorship of the work does not bear on my arguments, I will use the name on the original edition of *La nueva filosofía*, and the one used by Ildefonso Martínez: Oliva Sabuco.

6. On the construction of the past in classical antiquity, see Porter, "What Is 'Classical' about Classical Antiquity?"

7. Nicolas Masson de Morvilliers, "Espagne," in *Encyclopédie méthodique ou par ordre de matiéres.* On the controversy that ensued, see Herr, *The Eighteenth-Century Revolution in Spain,* 220–30, or for a more recent treatment, see Uzcanga Meinecke, *¿Qué se debe a España?*

8. Beneath the invective, there in fact existed a more complex reality, as demonstrated by Checa Beltran in *Demonio y modelo.*

9. Pimentel and Pardo-Tomás, "And yet we were modern."

10. Ibid., 135–36.

11. Navarro Brotons and Eamon, eds., *Mas allá de la leyenda negra: España y la revolución científica = Beyond the Black Legend: Spain and the Scientific Revolution.* Pimentel and Pardo-Tomás, "And yet we were modern," 137–38.

12. Latour, *We Have Never Been Modern.*

13. For one valuable corrective to this historiographic myopia, see Moreno Luzón, Archilés i Cardona, Molina Aparicio, and Balfour, *Construir España.* As the editors point out in their introduction, once theories of nationalism diverged from a top-down, state-driven model, more recent scholarship has been able to view "the Spanish case not as anomalous or exceptional, but rather as one within a wide array of European cases, each with its own peculiarities" (16).

14. Payne, *Spain,* 6.

15. Kagan, ed., *Spain in America,* 10. In fact, as José Alvarez Junco and Adrian Shubert remind us, in 1820 Spain was the first European country to fight for liberal freedom against reactionary absolutism. See Alvarez Junco and Shubert, eds., *Spanish History since 1808,* 6. And, as Stanley Payne goes on to point out, despite the vicissitudes of Spanish politics, "by 1923 Spain had lived under liberal parliamentary government for more years than had any other large continental European country, including France—no mean achievement for a 'historical failure'" (*Spain,* 143).

16. Kagan, "Prescott's Paradigm: American Historical Scholarship and the Decline of Spain," 425.

17. Peters, "Henry Charles Lea and the 'Abode of Monsters,'" 578.

18. Kagan, "Prescott's Paradigm," 446.

19. Alvarez Junco and Shubert, eds., *Spanish History since 1808,* 10. And, of course, the story was not limited to Europe, as Scott Eastman reminds us in *Preaching Spanish Nationalism across the Hispanic Atlantic.*

20. For comprehensive overviews of this work, see the introductions to the collections of essays edited by Alvarez Junco and Shubert, *Spanish History since 1808,* and *Nueva historia de la España contemporánea (1808–2018).*

21. Alvarez Junco and Shubert, *Nueva historia,* 38.

22. Michel Foucault famously viewed "subject formation" as a form of discipline rather than emancipation, and envisioned the prospect of the eventual "death of Man." See chapter 9 of his *The Order of Things.*

23. Caballé, "La biografía en España: primeras propuestas para la construcción de un canon," 109.

24. For a convincing defense of "historical biography," see Meister, "The Biographical Turn and the Case for Historical Biography."

25. Burdiel, "Historia política y biografía," 53. For an example of Burdiel's craft, see her *Isabel II: una biografía (1830–1904).*

26. Burdiel, "Historia política y biografía, 62.

27. See, for example, Renders and De Haan, *Theoretical Discussions of Biography: Approaches from History, Microhistory and Life Writing.*

28. Giovanni Levi paraphrased in Almagor, Ikonomou, and Simonsen, eds., *Global Biographies,* 12.

29. An important contribution to this rehabilitation can be found in Shortland and Yeo's edited collection, *Telling Lives in Science.* See also Miqueo and Ballester, eds., "Dossier: Biografías médicas, una reflexión historiográfica."

30. See chapter 4 of Shapin, *A Social History of Truth;* and Porter, *Doctor of Society: Thomas Beddoes and the Sick Trade in Late-Enlightenment England.*

31. Rosenberg, *Explaining Epidemics,* 215, qtd. in Hagner, "Scientific Medicine," 82.

32. Fuentes and Fernández Sebastián, "Liberalismo," in *Diccionario político y social del siglo XIX español,* 416, 418.

33. Ibid., 418.

34. Burdiel, "The Liberal Revolution, 1808–1843," 17.

35. Treatises such as Ramón López Mateos, *Pensamientos sobre la razón de las leyes derivada de las ciencias físicas ó sea sobre la filosofía de la legislación.*

36. Sirinelli, "De la demeure à l'agora," 385–86. Quoted in the introduction to Cabrera and Pro Ruiz, eds., *La creación de las culturas políticas modernas.*

37. For an overview of the development of the concept of "political culture," see Pérez Ledesma and Sierra's introduction to their *Culturas políticas,* 7–15.

38. On this process, see Rubio Pobes, "Patria y nación," in Cabrera and Pro Ruiz, eds., *La creación de las culturas políticas modernas,* 97–125.

39. Ibid., 103.

40. See chapter 12, "The Birth of the Liberal Tradition," in Herr, *The Eighteenth-Century Revolution in Spain,* 337–47. On this process see also chapter 4, "Historia nacional y memoria colectiva," in Álvarez Junco, *Mater Dolorosa.*

41. This discourse of "failure-ology" is examined in Roca Barea, *Fracasología.*

42. For a diagnosis of this scholarly neglect, see Alvarez Junco and Shubert's introduction to *Spanish History since 1808.*

1. Medical Politics and the Liberal Revolution

1. The term "guerrilla" stems from the unorthodox tactics adopted by the resistance to the Napoleonic invasion, although such tactics certainly predated the Peninsular War. See Laqueur, "The Origins of Guerrilla Doctrine."

2. On the international scope of these movements, see Anderson and Pols, "Scientific Patriotism," 98–99. Anderson and Pols provide as examples the German physician and social reformer Rudolf Virchow and his protégé, José Rizal, the Filipino independence leader.

3. Martykánová and Núñez-García, "Luces de España," 108.

4. López Piñero, "Las ciencias médicas en la España del siglo XIX," 206.

5. On this topic, see Guerra, "El exilio de médicos durante el siglo XIX." See also Llorens and Amorós, *Liberales y románticos.* For a more general analysis of the influence of exile in Spanish history, see Kamen, *The Disinherited.*

6. On the role of the military in the Liberal Revolution, see Boyd, "The Military in Politics."

7. A classic work on the Trienio is Gil Novales, *El trienio liberal.*

8. Artola, *La burguesía revolucionaria (1808–1874)*, 52.

9. López Piñero, "Las ciencias médicas en la España del siglo XIX," 210.

10. López Piñero, introduction to *M. Seoane, la introducción en España del sistema sanitario liberal, 1791–1870*, 15.

11. López Piñero, "Las ciencias médicas en la España del siglo XIX," 212.

12. Martínez's academic records are housed in the National Historical Archive in Madrid. See Martínez y Fernández, Universidades, 1225, exp. 8.

13. I use the capitalized English translations to distinguish the formal political parties from their underlying ideological tendencies. On the political contrasts between *moderados* and *progresistas,* see Romeo Mateo, "Lenguaje y política del nuevo liberalismo: moderados y progresistas, 1834–1845." For details on the formation of the Moderate and Progressive political parties, see Fernández Sarasola, *Los partidos políticos en el pensamiento español.* The scholarship on these political tendencies has tended to idealize the progresistas. For an alternative perspective, see Ramón Fernández, *La "década moderada" y la emergencia de la administración contemporánea.*

14. This is a simplified account of a complex situation. See Esdaile, *Spain in the Liberal Age,* 66–67.

15. López Piñero, "Las ciencias médicas en la España del siglo XIX," 219.

16. Rey González, "Clásicos de la psiquiatría del siglo XIX (IX)," 89.

17. Ibid. On the "edad de plata," see Laín Entralgo, *La edad de plata de la cultura española (1898–1936).*

18. Albarracín Teulón, "Las asociaciones médicas en España del siglo XIX," 120.

19. On this intermediate stage, see López Piñero, "Las ciencias médicas en la España del siglo XIX," 217–27.

20. Ibid., 219–20.

21. "Reglamento de la Sociedad Médico-Quirurgica de Emulación," 1839, BH AP 4 leg. 2, doc. 22, 1 (pagination mine): "Convencidos unánimente de que el unico objeto que nos reune es el de adquirir el conjunto de de conocimientos que cada uno tiene en particular."

22. "Economy" is used here in the technical medical sense of the bodily system as a whole.

23. Reglamento de la Sociedad Médico-Quirurgica de Emulación, 3–4.

24. Ildefonso Martínez y Fernández, "*Disertacion leída al Ateneo Médico-Quirurjico Matritense,*" 33 (pagination mine).

25. Ildefonso Martínez y Fernández, "Del influjo de lo físico en lo moral y vice-versa."

26. Fernández Sebastián, "Periodismo," in *Diccionario político y social del siglo XIX español,* 525.

27. Ibid., 526.

28. Miqueo, "Función de la prensa médica española en la difusión de la médecine physiologique (1820–1850)." On the rise of medical journalism in an Anglo-American context, see Bynum, Lock, and Porter, eds., *Medical Journals and Medical Knowledge.*

29. *La Verdad: Periódico de Medicina y Ciencias Auxiliares,* Madrid, September 22, 1847, 3. "Todas las ciencias encierran cosas inmutables y eternas como la divinidad, de quien emanan; pero tienen otras amovibles, perecederas y sujetas a los cambios y vicisitudes de los tiempos: ¿Quién disputará el derecho que a la prensa periódica asiste para representar ese interés de actualidad, ese flujo y reflujo de las ideas, esas mudanzas en las opiniones de los hombres?"

All translations are my own, unless otherwise noted. Ildefonso Martínez y Fernández, like many of his nineteenth-century contemporaries, wrote in a florid style. Consequently, in the interest of clarity I have translated loosely in some instances, reformulating grammatical structures, inserting punctuation, and eliding redundant verbiage. Also, the conventions dealing with spelling and accentuation were different in nineteenth-century Spanish; I have transcribed directly rather than attempting to modernize.

30. *La Verdad: Periódico de Medicina y Ciencias Auxiliares,* Madrid, September 22, 1847, 1. "El estado harto lastimoso por desgracia en que se halla en la actualidad la clase médica de España, la ninguna protección ni apoyo que merece . . . consecuencia precisa hasta cierto punto del total olvido e indiferencia con que la Sociedad los mira." This type of complaint was common throughout the nineteenth century. See Albarracín Teulón, "La profesión médica ante la sociedad española del siglo XIX," 303–16.

31. *La Verdad,* September 22, 1847, 2. "Nuestra profesión es un sacerdocio; como tal la miramos y, todos nuestros conatos se dirigirán a inculcar esta idea en el ánimo de nuestros jóvenes comprofesores. Pero este sacerdocio se parece en más de un concepto al religioso: paz, caridad, consuelo al infeliz, apoyo al desvalido, practican el párroco pobre y el médico de partido; intriga, cábalas, desprecio al que es inferior en la clase, ni una limosna al miserable, ni un consejo al que no puede pagar, esta es en general la conducta del médico de alto rango, canónigo prebendado lleno de goces y comodidades." This critique of elite physicians was not limited to Spain. See Williams, *The Physical and the Moral,* 69.

32. See, for example the issue of November 8, 1847.

33. See the final issue, September 22, 1848.

34. *Boletin de Medicina, Cirugía, y Farmacia* 71 (May 9, 1847): 151–53.

35. Ibid., 152: "visitando á troche y moche, haciendo tuertos, produciendo agravios, causando muertes, derribando enfermedades y produciendo peligros por do quiera."

36. Ibid.: "enemigos jurados de la salud."

37. Ibid.: "mas ávidos y chupones que sanguijuelas, solo sangrias sobre sangrias practican y bueno vaya . . . ah! triste, tristísima carrera la que sin freno mata y atormenta!"

38. Ibid.: "Entiéndase que al criticar aquí semejantes abusos no incluimos á los profesores de cirujía que honrados y caballeros solo asisten aquellos enfermos para quienes tienen autorización competente para visitarlos: conocemos muchos de ellos hombres probos y honrados y con ellos no trata la sátira de este artículo."

39. *Anales de Cirugía* 72 (May 16, 1847): 567. "¿No saben mejor que yo los redactores del Boletin que el tal Martínez no ha practicado bastante ni como médico ni como cirujano para que pueda juzgar a los demas? ¿Y como se vale de él para criticar y calificar de homicidas á tantos laboriosos profesores? Demencia completa fuera entrar en polémica con un ente tan ruin y miserable, con un loco digno de atar como Martínez el figurilla; en estas líneas me dirijo solo á los redactores del Boletin, pues solo á ellos los juzgo culpables en esta materia; de un loco como aquel nadie debe considerarse ofendido, lo que conviene es atarlo y tenerle lástima."

40. Ibid., 567n: "Le doy este nombre al doctor en medicina y cirugía don Ildefonso Martínez para que no se confunda con algun otro que hubiese de su mismo nombre. El Martínez á quien aludo es hijo de Pedro Martínez, tabernero y posadero en la posada de los Ángeles. Tiene una taberna . . . donde vive el doctor Martínez. Este por mas señas es de

estatura baja, cargado de espaldas, ancho de cara, mira ancho pero ve muy poco, gasta anteojos, es cuelli-corto, patizambo y muy grande hablador. . . . [E]ntiéndase que no trato de ridiculizar su físico, pues cada uno es como sus padres y Dios lo hicieron."

41. Ibid., 368: "se halla nada menos que todo un doctor en ciencias médicas respirando en una taberna y entonando al son de Baco esos infames dicterios?"

42. *El Boletín de Medicina, Cirugía, y Farmacia* 73 (May 23, 1847): 169: "Deploramos la necesidad en que nos vemos hoy de dar alguna contestación á lo que en el último número de los *Anales de Cirujía* se dice respecto á nuestro periódico; pero el silencio supondría convencimiento de una falta mas ó menos grave, y por eso no podremos pasar, siquiera lo destemplado y grosero del ataque, á los ojos de toda persona ilustrada, justificasen el silencio."

43. Ibid.: "que joven todavía, merece consideración y respeto de cuantos le trata: que tiene dadas infinitas pruebas de su instrucción y buen juicio para que hagan mella en su fama los dicterios de un anónimo."

44. Ibid., 169–70.

45. Ibid., 170.

46. See Albarracín Teulón, "La profesión médica ante la sociedad española del siglo XIX," 304.

47. *El Crisol* 1 (1855): 1: "[L]a angustiada frente se inunda de sudor frio al pasear nuestra vista por las melancolicas ruinas del edificio médico, de ese bello floron que tanta adorna al ramo de nuestros conocimientos, de este nutrido é importante vástago del árbol robusto del saber humano. ¡Oh nacion desgraciada que ves desplomarse insensiblemente el templo mas precioso que posees, la mayor garantía para tus aflicciones corporales bajo cuyo peso te doblegas á cada instante, y el mas poderoso consuelo de tu abatido espiritu!!!"

48. Ibid., 4–5: "un órgano en la prensa que fielmente abogue por su mejora positiva"; "el gobierno y los hombres de bien, sabedores de tamaños males, fijarán sus miradas en el horizonte de nuestro porvenir."

49. On this process of consolidation, see Jacobson and Moreno Luzón, "The Political System of the Restoration, 1875–1914."

50. On the uses of history in the creation of new political cultures in Spain during the nineteenth century, see Segarra, "La turbación de los tiempos."

51. Romero Alpuente, "Sucesión á la corona de España," 1–2 (pagination mine): "Cuando la España, hace mas de doce siglos, se bio abandonada de sus Reyes, y forzada á recobrar palmo á palmo su terreno usurpado por los Sarracenos, lo primero que recobró fue su soberania; y siendo ya antes electiba la corona, y legislador el pueblo, la parte de Aragon realizó, y afianzó estos derechos mas que la parte de Castilla; estableciendo para los reyes un genero de juramento, y para su vigilancia un Tribunal digno de un pueblo berdaderamente libre.

El juramento que los Aragoneses exigian á sus Principes, no es menos que el codigo de los derechos del Pueblo y las obligaciones de los Monarcas, pues era el siguiente: Vos, que no sois mas que cada uno de Nos, y Nos juntos somos mas que vos ¿jurais guardar nuestros fueros y libertades? "Si. juro respondia el Rey" y entonces concluian los Aragoneses con esta clausula inmortal, Pues si le guardais, sereis nuestro Rey; pero si non, non."

52. Ibid., 2: "El nombre del tribunal señalado para velar sobre su cumplimiento fué el de Justicia-Mayor de Aragon, y sus grandes facultades eran de oir las quejas, que los subditos daban contra el Rey."

53. Ibid., 3: "llegaron pronto á arrancar de la Corona la mas preciosa y brillante piedra de electiba, y reemplazarla con la peligrosa, y degradente de heretidaria."

54. Ibid., 4.

55. Ibid., 17.

56. Ibid., 15: "La fanatica e impolitica espulsion de los Moriscos, y Judios."

57. Martínez y Fernández, "Los partidos," 2 (pagination mine): "Una de las pretensiones mas frecuentes y repetidas de este partido es presentarse como el unico defensor de las antiguas creencias, de la vieja sociedad, como representante de la nacionalidad y tradicion historica."

58. Ibid.: "tachando a los liberales de innovadores, de revolucionarios, porque entonces nosotros les provaremos en que punto estuvieron los revolucionarios, de que filas salieron los innovadores, quienes fueron los que destruyeron los mas, las costumbres, los derechos y privilegios de los pueblos."

59. Ibid., 3: "un pueblo elegia el jefe del estado de entre los guerreros y sabios mas distinguidos y virtuosos, convocando en asamblea publico, ó sean Cortes, al clero, la nobleza ó patricios y la plebe; alli pues en aquel concurso en aquel concejo s votaba el candidato y se le investia con la autoridad suprema."

60. Ibid.: "Si el pueblo elegia el rey y la obligaba á que obedeciese las leyes y si no le destronaba; ¿que prueva mas ostenible de la soberania nacional? ¿donde queda pues el derecho divino?"

61. Ibid.: "la historia apoya el dogma de la soberania popular tan combatido por los realistas, y los revolucionarios é innovadores han sido aquellos que mal a venido, con aquella forma de gobierno se amaron para convertir segun la bella espresion de Romero Alpuente 'la brillante joya de electiva en la degradente de hereditaria.'"

62. Ibid., 4: "Las fuerzas de los condes y los duques, en monstruosa coalicion con las tropas alemanas hicieron sucumbir en Villalar esas doctrinas y sus valientes defensores." "Costo la nacion la perdida de todos sus fueros y libertades."

63. Ibid.: "No volvais la vista atrás comenzar desde el principio de este siglo y os contestaremos con la franqueza, provando la inutilidad de vuestras doctrinas y los perjuicios que han ocasionado y ocasionar pueden á la nacion."

64. Ibid.: "Llamanse serviles, realistas, aquellos individuos que apegados á las doctrinas despoticas de los reyes, reconocen en este al soberano, quien es dueño de vida y hacienda, pues aun cuando dicen que debe regir el estado segun las leyes, esto es lo mismo que manifestar segun su capricho, puesto que el rey reyna y gobierna, es decir, legisla y egecuta, sin otro poder ni ayuda que los que su santa voluntad llama á la formacion de las leyes, el las hace y las deroga sin que tengan otro derecho los ciudadanos que el de quejarse respetuosamente pero permaneciendo aquel sordo á los clamores."

65. Ibid., 5: "He aqui el absolutismo en su genuino sentido, he aqui la institucion de Carlos 10. Felipe 20. y demas reyes hasta nuestra regeneracion politica, pues si se nos digere que hubo cortes, consejo de castilla y consejo de estado manifestaremos que solo como cuerpos consultivos pero el veto real absoluto, es decir, la voluntad real podia reirse de los consejos y obrar lo que le diere la gana en favor de sus intereses."

66. Ibid.: "Los ignorantes, porque un educacion limitada y la direccion que pesó por tantos siglos sobre el pueblo, le han hecho creer que no debe ensayar otro sistema que el que tubo su padre ó un abuelo . . . Los egoistas, si bien conocen la bondad del sistema liberal le combaten

porque tienen intereses creados ó porque dependiendo de una de aquellas familias que por mucho tiempo monopolizaron los destinos de la nacion."

67. Ibid., 6: "son de dictamen que nadie puede ni debe escribir hablar enseñar ni pensar en contra del sistema establecido y de hacerlo asi castigarlos egemplar y severamente lo mismo á los pacificos que á los revolucionarios, de modo que su modo de tolerar se reduce á este formula, libertad para mi rey y altar, guerra á todos los que escriban en contra."

68. Ibid., 8: "sin prestigio porque no da ilusiones, sin verdad porque teme la discusion, sin justicia porque condena la razon, sin derechos porque uno solo posee todos."

69. On these developments, see Cruz, "The Moderate ascendancy, 1843–1868"; and Esdaile, *Spain in the Liberal Age*, 85–97.

70. Esdaile, *Spain in the Liberal Age*, 88–89. On these divisions, see also Bahamonde Magro and Martínez Martín, *Historia de España. Siglo XIX*, 250–54.

71. Martínez y Fernández, "Proyecto de una emancipación universal," 1 (pagination mine): "los Reyes se apoderaron de la clase media para hacerla servir á sus intereses como otro tiempo lejano se apoderaron de la aristocracia para destruir las libertades de los pueblos."

72. Ibid., 1–2: "advirtiendo con el mas profundo dolor que el abatimiento abyeccion é ignorancia de las masas depende de la falta de centralizacion en sus trabajos, de la desunion de sus esfuerzos, de la escasez de su ilustracion y mas que todo de su adoracion servil y esclava á idolos y personas mas bien enemigos que sinceras defensoras de los sacrosantos fueros de la humanidad, hemos determinado hacer un llamamiento general á todos los que se sientan con fuerzas para seguir en el precioso camino de las conquistas de la humanidad de la defensa de la humanidad, de la defensa de los hermanos todos en doctrina y principios, de la emancipa-cion universal."

73. Ibid., 1: "con los esfuerzos unidos de los obreros de la humanidad, de los libres de todos los paises, de todos los confines de todas las naciones, de todos los mundos."

74. Ibid., 3–4: "no hay naciones, no existen Alpes ni Pirineos, ni oceanos ni mediterraneo todos sois hermanos, todos obreros, todos participes de la desgracia ó la fortuna, de los bienes y los males porque todos os dirigis á un centro: solo la Emacipación, la Libertad."

75. Ibid., 6: "ciudadanos que gimen y padecen en la degradacion y miseria mientras unos cuantos zánganos absorben cuanto aquellos producen."

76. Ibid., 7: "Le formará una sociedad cuyo nombre sea la Emancipacion universal; cuyo objeto perenne y constante sea la mayor suma de libertad posible, la mejora intelectual, moral y material de la humanidad bajo formas constantes y uniformes."

77. For details on these societies, I am drawing on Castro Alfin, "The left: from liberalism to democracy," 79–90. See also, Castells, *La utopía insurreccional del liberalismo*.

78. Martínez, "Proyecto de una emancipación universal," 5: "A todos admitimos, á todos predicamos á todos escuchamos y á todos reunimos bajo nuestra bandera, carbonarios, ma-sones, comunistas, socialistas, comuneros, á todos llamamos al centro á la unidad á la doctrina."

79. Ibid., 8: "se puede acordar la paz ó la guerra, las elecciones, las combinaciones necesarias al grande objeto de la Emancipacion universal."

80. Ibid., 4: "Conquista grande y poderosa aquella en que entrando todos los pueblos lo mismo los unos que los otros, asi los viejos como los modernos, los paganos como los cristia-nos y en que unas mismas doctrinas universalicen unos principios puros y santos y un dia con las armas en la mano en una misma hora, á un mismo tiempo, dirigidos á un fin, con iguales tendencias á derrocar el imperio de la usurpacion y á establecer el de la igualdad de derechos

el de la conquistas filosoficas, de la tolerancia, de la libertad y mutua enlaze de intereses de los unos pueblos con los otros como hijos todos de un padre comun."

81. Martínez y Fernández, "Democracia, o El Porvenir," 1 (pagination mine): "En medio de nuestras mas apuradas epocas, en esos periodos de crisis por [los] que ha pasado el pueblo español desde el principio de este siglo, en esos movimientos y convulsiones revolucionarias, aun no ha aparecido entre nosotros un periodico que se dedique a predicar á enseñar y propagar los principios de la libertad y las demasías de la tirania, sin personalizarlos, elevandose solo al sublime campo de las concepciones y sostiendo lo que unicamente puede sostenerse, a saber la pureza de los principios."

82. Ibid., 8: "no usará de otras armas que la razon y alguna vez el sarcasmo pero siempre con el decoro debido á los que sustentan como base la tolerencia con todas las opiniones y el respeto con todas las personas. . . . Entrará en polemica de principios con los periodicos contrarios en opiniones, porque no teme las doctrinas que contienen otros principios porque los cree erroneos é insubsistentes y el crisol de la discusion hara resaltar los principios democraticos tanto como el sol brilla en medio de las densas nieblas de un dia de invierno."

83. Ibid., 5: "podréis con las armas de la discusión y tolerancia hacer de un enemigo un amigo, de un absolutista un republicano."

84. Ibid., 4: "es el interes de los mas contra los menos, de los derechos contra los privilegios, de la honrradez contra la desmoralizacion, de la economia contra el despulsamiento del orden popular contra la anarquia gubermental, de la libertad contra la tirania, de la igualdad ante la ley contra la monopolio de los ricos, de la ilustracion contra la ignorancia, . . . es en fin el triunfo de los principios evangelicos y de las doctrinas del hombre Dios contra los principios de monopolio y gobernacion de los fariseos politicos, es pues, ultimamente la causa de la justicia de los pueblos, contra los intereses y usurpaciones de las testas coronadas."

85. Ibid., 7, 8: "un verdadero comunismo de ideas, pensamientos y doctrinas"; "levantar de los escombros y el envilecimiento la libertad moribunda."

86. Ibid., 6: "Si sufreis persecuciones por la defensa de vuestros principios, no por eso abandoneis la empresa, sufrid con valor las inculpaciones y *si son relativas a vuestros principios* no seáis tan pusilanimes que neguéis un bondad y oportunidad, tened valor, en sostener los en la adversidad que el martirologio es la base mas solida de las doctrinas del porvenir."

87. Ibid.: "Si os abruman con contribuciones que no estén votadas por los mandatarios de la nacion, negadlas y formad asociados una muralla que solo pueda romper la violencia, porque los medios violentos traen en pos de si la ruina de los gobiernos que la perpetran."

88. Martínez y Fernández, *Espejo del verdadero médico,* 158.

89. Esdaile, *Spain in the Liberal Age,* 53.

90. Ibid. See also Ruiz Torres, "Modelos sociales del liberalismo español."

91. Sierra, "La cultura politica en el estudio del liberalismo y sus conceptos de representación," 233–36, 253.

92. Barnosell, "God and Freedom: Radical Liberalism, Republicanism, and Religion in Spain, 1808–1847," 42. And these religious currents were not limited to Spain, but rather part and parcel of revolutionary political cultures throughout Southern Europe, as Maurizio Isabella demonstrates in part IV of *Southern Europe in the Age of Revolutions.*

93. Martínez y Fernández, "Proyecto de una emancipación universal," 11–12.

94. López Piñero, "Las ciencias médicas en la España del siglo XIX," 218.

2. Spanish Medicine and the Science of Man

1. Foucault describes this development in chapter 2 of *The Birth of the Clinic*.

2. The classic work on Virchow is Ackerknecht, *Rudolf Virchow, Doctor, Statesman, Anthropologist*. See also McNeely, *"Medicine on a Grand Scale": Rudolf Virchow, Liberalism, and the Public Health*.

3. This process has been detailed in section 1 of Arquiola and Montiel, *La corona de las ciencias naturales*, 5–73.

4. Benavente Barreda, "Sensualismo," 265–66. See also Navarro and Gisbert, "La recepción del sensualismo."

5. Gracia Guillén, "Ideología y ciencia clínica en la España de la primera mitad del siglo XIX," 237.

6. Staum, *Cabanis*, 4.

7. Cabanis, *On the Relations between the Physical and Moral Aspects of Man*, 33.

8. Ibid., 39. On the changing definitions of "metaphysics," see Reed, *From Soul to Mind*, 32–33.

9. Cabanis, *On the Relations between the Physical and Moral Aspects of Man*, 116: "In order to have an accurate idea of the operations from which thought results, it is necessary to consider the brain as a special organ designed especially to produce it, as the stomach and the intestines are designed to operate the digestion."

10. Ginsburg and Jablonka, *The Evolution of the Sensitive Soul*, 44.

11. Jacyna, "Medical Science and Moral Science," 119.

12. Staum, "Cabanis and the Science of Man."

13. Williams, *The Physical and the Moral*, 3.

14. Ibid.

15. Staum, *Cabanis*, 205.

16. On Alibert, see Williams, *The Physical and the Moral*, 122–36.

17. Novella, "La medicina de las pasiones en la España del siglo XIX," 466–67.

18. For background on Monlau, see Campos Marín, *Monlau, Rubio, Giné: curar y gobernar*. See also Vázquez García, "Un gobierno que se limita a sí mismo: La biopolítica liberal clásica," in *La invención del racismo*, 183–221.

19. Monlau y Roca, *Elementos de higiene pública*, 723–24: "Los pueblos, como los individuos, tienen sus necesidades; y los pueblos, como los individuos, tienen, por consiguiente, sus pasiones. La pasion no es mas que una necesidad exagerada, violenta, que tiraniza al hombre, que le avasalla, que perterba su razon, que hace enfermar su cuerpo. Y las pasiones, consideradas en las masas de individuos, no son tampoco mas que necesidades violentamente satisfechas ó mal reprimidas, que perturban el órden público, constityen la corrupcion de costumbres, y son el mas terrible obstáculo para la buena educacion de los pueblos." On Monlau's adaptation of French *idéologie*, see Sánchez Villa, *Entre materia y espíritu*, 122–26.

20. Ibid., 724: "Una sociedad en la cual se noten tales vicios y tales delitos, está necesariamente enferma, corrompida, es víctima de las pasiones, necesariamente *padece:* los preceptos higiénicos, que son tambien los de la religion y de la moral, han sido en ella conculcados; y fuerza es aplicar un remedio si se quiere que la corrupcion no llegue á producir caos."

21. Ibid., 736: "Sin trabajo nada fructifique; la riqueza no es mas que el trabajo acumulado;

y la naturaleza hizo al hombre el rey del universo, bajo la expresa condicion de trabajar. La pereza es contraria á las leyes, á la moral, al órden público, y tambien á la salud del individuo. . . . La pobreza es compañera de la pereza, dice el libro de los Proverbios; y el bienestar es el fruto de la actividad."

22. Ibid., 867: "Por último, la Medicina política, además de una Administration especial, además de un código sanitario y de reglamentos adecuados, y además de los auxilios de un publicacion periódica, necesita tambien tener intérpretes en el profesorado. . . . Solo con estas medidas será hacedero el poner en práctica las reglas de la Higiene, y el disponerse para llevar á cabo las mejoras ó reformas que cada año irán demandando los progresos de la civilizacion."

23. Ronzón, *Antropología y antropologías*, 224.

24. *Boletín de medicine, cirugía, y farmacia* 8 (July 24, 1834): 57: "En efecto, desde Hipócrates hasta Copérnico, Galileo, Loche, Linneo, Fourcroi, Cubier, no hay parte alguna del saber humano que no deba á los médicos los mas grandes servicios, estendiéndose su importancia y necesidad á la moral, á la política, y á la legislación de los pueblos."

25. Ibid., 58: "que estudia sus pasiones y sus vicios, enfermedades morales solo bien conocidas y curables, cuando se conoce al hombre físico."

26. Ibid.: "La educacion de la juventud, cuyo principal resorte debería ser la recta dirección de sus hábitos y costumbres, enseñándoles á dominar sus pasiones é inclinaciones, y manifestándoles los deberes que los unen con los demás hombres, no se estudia sin duda fuera de la consideración del hombre físico."

27. Ibid.: "Se cree de una inmensa extension la ciencia del hombre, y lo es sin duda, porque ella lo conserva, lo educa, lo gobierna, pero siempre debe comenzarse por conocerlo para conservarlo, para dirigirlo y para gobernarlo." This language immediately brings to mind the work of Foucault, who comments in *The Birth of the Clinic*, "One began to conceive of a generalized presence of doctors whose intersecting gazes form a network and exercise at every point in space, and at every moment in time, a constant, mobile, differentiated supervision" (31).

28. *Boletín de Medicina, Cirugía, y Farmacía* 8 (July 24, 1834): 58: "El bien social no puede tener lugar sino de una manera adecuada á las localidades de las naciones, es decir, al espíritu y á las disposiciones físicas de los pueblos."

29. Ibid.: "Conozcamos los hombres, repito, para dirigirlos."

30. Ibid.: "Una falsa igualdad entre las clases."

31. Ibid., 58–59: "He aquí por qué las autoridades principales, tanto políticas como religiosas de las provincias, debieran hacer un profundo estudio de sus habitantes, y he aquí también por qué las autoridades centrales de la nacion deben precisamente tener á su lado representantes instruidos que, identificados con cada provincia en particular, puedan ilustrarles." Foucault, in turn, describes his conception of "biopower" as "a power that exerts a positive influence on life, that endeavours to administer, optimize, and multiply it, subjecting it to precise controls and comprehensive regulations" (*The History of Sexuality* 1: 137).

32. Varela de Montes et al., *Ensayo de antropología*. See for example, Fabra Soldevila, *Filosofía de la legislación natural fundada en la antropología o en el conocimiento de la naturaleza del hombre y de sus relaciones con los demás seres*. For an exhaustive list of similar works, see Sánchez Villa, *Entre materia e espíritu*, 113n221.

33. See, for example, Novella, *La ciencia del alma,* and by the same author, *El discurso psico-patológico de la modernidad;* See also part I of Sánchez Villa, *Entre materia y espíritu.*

34. See Gútiez, "Ildefonso Martínez, amigo y bibliotecario de Gallardo."

35. Gallardo, "Sensaciones," 64–77, and "Sentidos," 93–100. On Martínez's relationship with Gallardo, see Gútiez, "Ildefonso Martínez, amigo y bibliotecario de Gallardo."

36. Gallardo y Blanco, *Don Bartolomé José Gallardo, 1776–1852. Estudio Bibliográfico,* 29: "El hombre debe ser el blanco de todas las Ciencias; el hombre lo es especialísimamente de la Medicina.—¿De qué nos servirian las mas exquisitas investigaciones sobre las propiedades de los cuerpos, si no nos prestasen ayuda para conocer mejor el humano, y de consiguiente para aumentar nuestros deleytes, y evitarnos los males físicos de que está rodeada sin cesar nuestra máquina, en fuerza de su continuo choque con todos los elementos? Pues si de las Ciencias Físicas pasamos á las Intelectuales y Morales, estas nada son sin el auxilio de la Medicina. La Moral no puede hacer adelantamientos sin que los haga ántes la Ideología, y esta no dará un paso, si no se apoya en la Fisiología. Jamas se ha visto tan patente esta verdad, como ahora que se ha hecho casi de moda el estudio de la correlation del hombre físico y moral."

37. Ildefonso Martínez y Fernández, "*Disertacion leída al Ateneo Médico-Quirúrjico Ma-tritense,*" 1 (pagination mine): "La ciencia que se ocupa del reyno humanal . . . en sus relaciones fisicias, intelectuales y morales, es Antropologia, esto es, ciencia del hombre."

38. Ibid., 2: "[Se]gun Cabanis, quien mejor conocerá, el ser intelectual y moral? A quien que conozca mejor sus necesidades, como producto de su organizacion, y los medios de satisfacerlas: y esto supuesto. Este conocimiento de donde viene? Del juego que desempeñan nuestros organos, de sus alteraciones y modificaciones, por ciertos y determinados agentes y de consiguiente de los medios que la naturaleza pone en acion, que es justamente lo que examina la Medicina."

39. Ibid.: "El estudio mas propio del hombre, dice Pope, es el hombre mismo" porque solo conociendose el hombre asi, puede conocer a los demas. Desde la mas remota antigüedad, se conoció esta maxima, que se hallaba inscripta en el frontispicio del templo de Delphos, con no menos claridad que consticion "Nosce ipsum" Maxima que debiera estar gravada en el corazon de todos los hombres, como el principio de la felicidad social, como fuente de los bienes humanos, que debe transmitirse de generacion en generacion, de pueblo en pueblo, de gente en gente, para que de este modo fuese tan eterna y respetada como eterna la existencia del universo."

40. Ibid., 3–4: "Nada es mas natural, en el hombre, que tener pasiones y deseos; . . . Las pasiones humanas, son la expresión de las necesidades de su ser, como lo es el hambre y otras sensaciones; pues son necesarias . . . para la conservacion del organismo."

41. Ibid., 5: "el hombre que cultiva sus facultades inteletcuales, y descuida el regimen de sus pasiones, es el mas desgraciado de todos los mortales."

42. Ibid., 6: "El hombre como familia, consigue su felicidad domestica, sabiendo lo que nosotros valemos y apreciar en su justo valor las propiedades que los demas miembros de la familia tienen, de modo que conociendonos á nosotros mismos, y dirigiendo á los demas por sus inclinaciones naturales, modificada por una buena educacion, tendremos que dar á cada uno aquella carrera, arte ú oficio, que mas en relacion esté con sus facultades fisicas, intelec-tuales, y morales."

43. Ibid.: "Y efectivamente no pudiera menos de ser asi porque en suma que es la sociedad?

No es otra cosa que la reunion de individuos, con sus temperamentos, habitos, costumbres, idiosincracias y suos. Y si esto es asi, claro está que se deben mejorar los individuos, para reformar las sociedades, en una palabra si queremos mejorar los gobiernos, advirtamos que es preciso empezar la reforma por nosotros mismos."

44. Ibid.: "El despotismo paternal hecha los cimientos al despotismo social." The original quote is from Volney, *The Ruins*, 33.

45. On Volney's influence in Spain, see Castro Alfín, "Los ideólogos en España."

46. Hervás y Panduro, *Carta del abate Don Lorenzo Hervás*, 13: "El padre por naturaleza y razon es superior no solamente á los hijos, mas también á la consorte; porque si no lo fuera, en una familia tendriamos la monstruosidad de dos cabezas. La madre, sujeta al padre, es ciertamente superior á los hijos; y entre estos el primogénito se hace respetable á los demás hermanos, porque es el que mas inmediatamente sucede al padre." For this discussion of contributions to conservative political culture in nineteenth-century Spain, I am drawing on sources and ideas presented by Cabrera in "El sujeto de la política," 37–67.

47. Villanueva, *Catecismo del estado según los principios de la religión*, 22: "Los hijos de Adan heredamos de nuestro padre el amor á la independencia, de donde nació su pecado. La subordinación corrige y refrena en nosotros este afecto, y nos preserva de sus daños. Esta subordinación no puede establecerse ni asegurarse, á no haber autoridad y poder que la haga observar. Por eso no es duradera la sociedad donde unos hombres no están sujetos á otros. La independencia y la anarquía conspiran á la ruina y disolución de la sociedad. No hay sociedad donde cada qual sin temor de freno ni de castigo da rienda á sus pasiones y antojos."

48. Ibid., 134–35. "Habíanse menester unos á otros los miembros del cuerpo político, no menos que los del cuerpo natural: pero les faltaba el verdadero amor que impele al hombre al sufrimiento de la agena miseria, y al socorro de la agena necesidad, y á dar parte á los otros los frutos de su propio trabajo."

49. Freyre de Castrillón, *Contra el contrato social*, 8–9. "la multitud, abandonada á la se- ducción de intereses y pasiones particulares, tuerce el sentido de las leyes; vicia las partes más sanas de la administración; cede el lugar del zelo á la fuerza y á la inteligencia, ; y como una ponzoña secreta que sofoca los primeros movimientos de la vida, destruye los principios que conservan la acción y orden del Estado" (quoted by Cabrera, "El sujeto de la política," 45).

50. Novella, *La ciencia del alma*, 147–48. See also, Sánchez Villa, *Entre materia y espíritu*, 51.

51. Martínez y Fernández, "Disertacion leída al Ateneo Médico-Quirurjico Matritense," 34: "Criar un niño es servirse de sus disposiciones naturales, de su temperamento, de su sensib- ilidad, de sus necesidades y sus pasiones para modificarle ó formarle segun se debe monstran- dole los que debe amar ó temer y enseñarle los medios de conseguirlo ó evitarlo."

52. Ibid., 35: "Y vosotros, ministros de la religion, á quien estubo tanto tiempo confiada la educacion de la jubentud, dejad de poner trabas al entendimiento humano, abandonad á algunos de vosotros cohermanos, que trabajan encesantemente para introducir el despotismo y la tirania. . . . Los gobiernos despoticos temen mas una buena educacion, que todas las armas que se les cuestan, y segun la espresion del tirano Licinio la educacion y las ciencias son la sarcoma de los Estados."

53. Ibid., 39: "Pero una de las pasiones que debe de educarse con predileccion es, el sentimiento mas noble y de mayor interes para las sociedades á saber el Amor Patrio, que es la unica pasion que voy a analizar en particular tanto por su utilidad como por presentar á la consideracion de mis dignos consocios alguna cosa que les pueda ser agradables."

54. Ibid., 40: "Donde hay Patria tal cual la hemos descrito hay una pasion, un sentimiento exaltado y sublime producido por el instinto mas bien que por la reflexion que prefiere en todas ocasiones el interes general al individual, fuente eterna de heroismo y de prodigios politicos y el resorte mas poderoso para elebar y conservar los estados, pasion que se siente mas bien que se define que se inspira y no se esplican, sentimiento en fin, que dice mas con una sola accion á un alma virtuosa que todas las espresiones de los filosofos, que arrebata nuestra admiracion, exalta nuestra envidia y arrastra despues tras sí el vivo deseo de la imitacion." Martínez is quoting here from Manuel José Quintana, "Reflexiones sobre el patriotismo," *Semanario Patriótico*, no. 3 (September 15, 1808): 48.

55. Ibid., 43–44: "El patriotismo semejante al fuego, á la luz, á la electricidad á los demas grandes agentes de la naturaleza, es el mismo para todos los hombres." Here, again, Martínez is borrowing from Quintana. See "Reflexiones sobre el patriotismo," 50-51.

56. Ibid., 46: "borrar de las paginas de la historia la degradante y perfida maxima Francesa de que: 'La España mas bien pertenece á Africa que á Europa en el mapa politico de las naciones, pues los españoles son por naturaleza esclavos.'" Contrary to the opinion of Martínez, the French were not unanimously dismissive of Spanish culture. See Checa Beltran, *Demonio y modelo.*

57. Martínez y Fernández, "Disertacion leída al Ateneo Médico-Quirurjico Matritense," 47: "[A]ntes que la Francia tubiera un Voltaire y un Lafonten tubimos nosotros un Calderon y un Lope de Vega, que antes de un Montesquieu hubo en España un Alfonso el savio."

58. Ibid., 49–50: "Vosotros, Franceses, que en otros tiempos disteis á las naciones oprimidas la señal de la libertad, quereis, voltarios é insensatos, que ahora [os] ayuden á llevar la coyunda de la esclavitud."

59. Ibid., 50: "A vosotros dignos consocios mios, á vosotros imitadores de Esculapio, toca la epoca de la regeneracion social de nuestra Patria, en que cimentados los principios morales sobre la naturaleza del hombre podais formar una hera de honor y gloria de la desgraciada España! Estudiad, en paz, si estudiad en paz; que ya feneció el imperio del terror, que con las armas de la ignorancia, protegia el error en unos, la hipocracia en otros, el fanatismo y la supersticion en muchos. Renació ya el imperio de la Santa libertad (que sin permitir el libertinage ni la irreligion) busca la verdad y la protégé donde la encuentra."

60. Ibid., 51: "Armemonos, pues contra la corrupcion moral, libremos nuestra Patria de los brazos onerosos del despotismo y la tirania oponiendo por antemural nuestros debiles pechos arrastrando muerte gloriosa, libertando la sociedad de manos perdidas y serviles, podrán nuestros nombres ser borrados de la lista de los vivos, pero jamas de la memoria de los hombres sensatos y virtuosos, en quienes un sentimiento de amor patria haga batir el corazon."

61. Martínez y Fernández, "Del influjo de lo físico en lo moral y vice-versa," 2: "la corta consideracion social que han tenido los medicos para con las naciones y sus gobiernos."

62. Ibid., 3–4: "El influjo del lo moral en lo fisico y vice-versa, es un asunto de la mayor importancia y una de aquellas cuestiones que naturalmente se presentará a la vista de quien contempla el augusto soberano del universo, el hombre, ese ser el mas perfecto de la escala animal."

63. Ibid., 5: "aparecieron sabios observadores y manifestaron la influencia que lo fisico tiene en lo moral, llevando la medicina á la filosofia. . . ."

64. Ibid., 12–13: "¿Pues quien sino los medicos que conocen el ser fisico y el moral, en cuanto nos es dado alcanzar este conocimiento, pueden ocuparse de este asunto? ¿Serán los

teologos, con sus vanas sugestiones, con sus enrredosas disputas é incomprensibles misterios? ¿Serán los filosofos, embebidos en sus altas especulaciones, ó serán los matematicos ocupados de problemas y calculos, en que se pierde inutilmente su raciocinio?"

"Con hechos, pues, debe contestarse á hechos, y pudiendo ascender de los hechos á los teorias, como pueden hacerlo los medicos, tendremos lugar de ver fomando un dia, el cuadro ideal y el retrato mas perfecto pulido y completo del hombre fisico y moral."

65. Ibid., 31.

66. Ibid., 32.

67. Ibid., 32–33: "[I]lustres consocios, no desmayeis su momento en vuestros grandes proyectos, no os dejeis arrastrar tampoco de las pasiones mas mezquinas, consolidad el edificio que vosotros mismos levantaisteis; edificad sobre esos cimientos solidos, el alcazar de la Medicina Patria, y merecereis bien de ella, y de los hombres en quienes todavia circule la sangre de los Laras, Pelayos y Zuñigas; y cuyas almas puedan elevarse aun á los heroicos hechos de Numancia y de Sagunto, antes que consentir, que en vuestros generosos corazones penetre la argucia y la envidia. Si, consocios el conocimiento que tengo de vosotros, me hace aseverar vuestros juramentos, y me manifiesta que sola la . . . emulacion, es nuestra bandera y bajo la cual pelearemos sin abandonar la jamas, hasta rendir el ultimo suspiro."

68. Cabanis, *On the Relations between the Physical and Moral Aspects of Man,* 33.

69. Rigoli, "The 'Novel of Medicine,'" 77, 88.

70. Martínez y Fernández, "Tratado de fisiología #2," 1r: "La ciencia que nos enseña á conocer al hombre en su estado natural es la que nos ocupa y se conoce con el nombre de Fisiologia. Ciencia no menos util al naturalista, que al legislador, al economista que al literato, al sacerdote que al ciudadano, y finalmente á todas las clases de la Sociedad. Al naturalista le conviene proporcionandole medios, si posible fuese, de perfeccionar la naturaleza misma; al legislador marcándole el camino que debe seguir en la imposición de las leyes mas propias al carácter y felicidad de la sociedad á quien pertenece; al economista, dictándole el areglo interior de la corporación que representa; al literato, amenizandole con descripciones sencillas que representen las costumbres y placeres mas filantrópicos á todas las clases; al sacerdote, único director en nuestra infancia, imprimiéndole los sentimientos mas sanos y virtuosos; al ciudadano, indicándole la importancia que los derechos sociales egercen sobre él, diferenciandole del hombre idiota y salvage; y finalmente á todas las clases, para cumplir con sus deberes . . . para ser útiles á la sociedad a que pertenecen; con sus pasiones para estimularlas cuando son buenas, y reprimirlas cuando son malas. Siendo esta la utilidad de la Fisiología, acaso no seria dificil demonstrar como principio: Que la ruina de los Ymperios y grandes naciones dependen de la ignorancia en que yacen los miembros que las constituyen respecto de esta ciencia tan util a los derechos sociales y á la libertad, como á la felicidad y bienestar de la Patria."

71. Ibid., 39v: "las instituciones morales tienen su origen en la naturaleza del hombre y en su misma organizacion ya dependan de la vida individual ya de la especial, en cuyo primer caso atienden estas instituciones á la conservacion del individuo y en el segundo á la de la especie; y como estas sean los principios generales de la legislacion hé aqui de que modo la fisiologia es la dominadora de las leyes; porque no se puede concebir como se forma sin estos dos requisitos que indudablemente forman el atributo esencial del estado social; pues si el hombre no tiende á conservar á si mismo ni a su especie no se puede concebir la vida ni menos la mutua la relacion de los diferentes individuos."

72. Ibid., 40r: "la misma moral tiene su origen en la naturaleza del hombre á causa de la ley de sensibilidad."

73. Ibid., 40v: "la union constituye su fuerza."

74. Ibid., 5v: "esta fuerza para observar la naturaleza, surcar los mares, cultivar la tierra, estraer de las entrañas de esta los metales, dominar los animales mas feroces y finalmente para que contribuyera á nuestra felicidad por medio de la legislacion."

75. Ibid., 40v: "y ved aqui como la opinion publica alcanza hasta á los Reyes sobre sus tronos, obligandolos á contenerse bajo los limites de una autoridad regular, dependiendo todo esto del conocimiento del hombre ó sea de su fisiologia."

76. On this tendency, see Torrecilla, *España al revés,* 40–48.

77. Martínez y Fernández, "Compendio biográfico-bibliografico de la fisiologia," 14 (pagination mine).

78. Ibid.

79. Ibid., 9: "pero no los filosofos los hombres humanitarios y filantropicos que no ven en los hombres de distintas opiniones religiosas mas que sus hermanos seres enteramente semejantes y cuya diversa religion no los puede separar."

80. Ibid., 19: "los mas atroces martirios para los desgraciados que cayesen en ojeriza del clero."

81. Ibid., 25: "Muchas cosas han influido en este siglo para que las ciencias no progresasen y mucho mas aun la fisiologia esa rama de la medicina que es la que mas libertad necesita para sus discusiones se encuentra ahogada por el despotismo inquisitorial pues se tenia que buscar un mecenas de valia en la corte un santo un clerigo un obisbo ó tal vez un familiar de la Ynquisicion á fin de poder publicar sus doctrinas cubriendolas siempre con el velo del misticismo religioso y apoyandose en textos de los A.A. sagrados."

82. Ibid., 19: "la aplicacion de la Anatomia á la teologia moral, á la escultura y á la politica."

83. Arrizabalaga, "The Ideal Medical Practitioner," 68.

84. Redondo, "La métaphore du corps de la République à travers le traité du médicine Jerónimo Merola," 43.

85. On Merola's use of the body politic metaphor, see Vicente-Pedraz, "Cuerpo y política en la república original (1587), de Jerónimo Merola," 239–63.

86. Merola, *República original,* 120r–v: "En vn reyno gouierna vn Rey, y tiene baxo de si subditos que le obedecen con toda razon y ley: y a estos le tiene fomentados con justicia, hecha con toda blandura, y mezclada con mucha misercordia, y tine cabe si Principes y grandes, por cuyo ministerio gouierna, valiendose dellos en tiemps de paz y de guerra, y como tales les alça de estado, con mercedes y con honrras, cometiendoles sus vezes y acciones. Esto passa muy al pie de la letra en el humano cuerpo, el quel viene ser regido y gouernado por naturaleza, como por su Rey, y tan justo, que a ninguna parte haze agrauio, ni le quita lo que es suyo, antes de siempre, y le esta influyendo calor y espiritus, y la esta fomentando de manera que de buena gana la obedecen y la reconocen en paz y en guerra (digo en el tiempo de salud y de la enfermedad)."

87. Redondo, "La métaphore du corps de la République à travers le traité du médicine Jerónimo Merola," 50.

88. Merola, *República original,* 256r–v: "los que forman en si opiniones baxas y pagizas, e indignas de hombre Philosopho, an de ser contados entre los plebeos y populares, sean

ellos los que fueren Reyes Duques o Doctores, y por el contrario seran computados entre los mas baxo estado vienen a esmerarse tanto en sus costumbres, y opiniones, que dexan atras a muchos Principes, y hombres de auentajada fortuna."

89. Ibid., 256v: "medir a los hombres, por lo que mejor y de mas valor ay en ellos, que son las cosas del animo y entendimeinto, y no por lo que antojadiza fortuna les a dado."

90. Arrizabalaga, "The Ideal Medical Practitioner," 74–80.

91. Jorge Enríquez, *Retrato del perfecto médico,* 110.

92. For an examination of the details surrounding the Inquisition's censorship of Huarte, see Giglioni, "Between Galen and St Paul," and Arrizabalaga, "Huarte de San Juan y la censura inquisitorial en la España de Felipe II." Arrizabalaga's article is also one of the few recent pieces to mention Ildefonso Martínez y Fernández's editions of the *Examen* and the *Nueva filosofía.*

93. One year after the initial 1845 printing of Martínez edition of the *Examen,* a reprint was issued. Unless otherwise noted, all subsequent citations are from Martínez's 1846 edition of Huarte and and his 1847 edition of Sabuco.

94. On these parallels between Huarte and Sabuco, see Sumillera "Political Medicine in Early Modern Spain," 429–31.

95. Serés, "Huarte de San Juan: de la 'naturaleza' a la 'política,'" 80.

96. Sabuco, *New Philosophy,* 44, quoted by Sumillera in "Political Medicine in Early Modern Spain," 431.

97. In an editor's note to the *Examen,* Martínez explicitly situates Huarte in terms of the science of man. See *Examen,* 39n1.

98. Cabanis, *On the Relations Between the Physical and Moral Aspects of Man,* 236.

99. Ibid., 236–37.

100. Martínez y Fernández, "Del influjo de lo moral en lo físico y vice-versa," 25: [P]or los hombres existe el mundo abstracto y de las especulaciones, á que no puede remontarse la muger."

101. Ibid.: "son timidas, astutas, celosas, inconstantes, compasivas, caritativas y supersticiosas."

102. Martín Araguz, "Spanish Brain Science and Philosophy of Mind in the Time of Cervantes," 16.

103. *Examen,* 276: "las hembras por razon de la frialdad y humedad de su sexo, no pueden alcanzar ingenio profundo; solo vemos que hablan con alguna apariencia de habilidad en materias livianas y fáciles, con términos comunes y muy estudiados; pero metidas en letras no pueden aprender mas que un poco latin, y esto por ser obra de la memoria. De la cual rudeza no tienen ellas la culpa, sino que la frialdad y humedad que las hizo hembras, estas mismas calidades hemos probado atras que contradicen al ingenio y habilidad."

104. Ibid., 404. "las mugeres son inhábiles para el mayor número de ciencias, y esto no solo depende de su educacion moral y política, sino de su propia organizacion, diferente en mucho á la del hombre."

105. Martínez, "Del influjo de lo físico en lo moral y vice-versa," 26: "Todo esto debe tomarse en un sentido general, pues en el absoluto no es cierto . . . luego seguramente que hay excepciones bastante considerables."

106. Pomata, introduction to Nantes Barrera, *The True Medicine,* 10.

107. *La Verdad,* September 22, 1847, 4: "hemos convenido en ser corteses comenzando por la obra de una dama que honra nuestra literatura."

108. Sabuco, *Nueva filosofía,* 75: "[T]an elocuente como es la autora en castellano tanto lo es en latin, por lo que no es estraño que cuanto mas se estudie esta produccion, se convenza uno mas y mas de que fué un hombre y no una muger el escritor de esta bellísima obra."

109. Ibid., 9–10: "Difícil es creer que una muger haya podido ser tan périta en las ciencias." In fact, as Gianna Pomata has demonstrated, Oliva Sabuco's erudition did not go unremarked upon at the time. She was lauded by Cristóbal de Acosta in his *Tratado en loor de las mugeres* (*Treatise in Praise of Women*), written before the publication of the *New Philosophy,* although not published until 1592. See Sabuco, *The True Medicine,* 23–30.

110. See Vintró and Waithe, "*¿Fue Oliva o fue Miguel?*" and, by Waithe and Vintró, "Postumously Plagiarizing Oliva Sabuco." For Pomata's response, see the introduction to *The True Medicine.*

111. Vintró and Waithe, "*¿Fue Oliva o fue Miguel?*" 84: "Hay quien dice que esta obra no fue de muger, yo estoy persuadido á que sí, el soberano a quien se dedicó fué demasiado porque grave y circunspecto para que en materia tan importante y seria nadie se atreviese á hablarle disfrazado." In an error of attribution, the WorldCat database incorrectly lists Martín Martínez, rather than Ildefonso Martínez, as the editor of the 1847 version.

112. *La Verdad,* September 22, 1847, 4.

113. Sabuco, *Nueva filosofía,* 79: "una edicion filosófica, mas que una simple reimpresion."

114. Martykánová and Núñez García, "Ciencia, patria y honor," 49. On "Romantic masculinity," see also Sierra, "Política, romanticismo y masculinidad."

115. *El Siglo Médico* 31 (August 6, 1854): 241: "Creemos escusado insistir en la necesidad y conveniencia de que las clases médicas tomen una gran parte en la reorganizacion politica y social que va á verificarse. . . ." "destruir el error en que el pueblo se hallaba de que los médicos solo sirven para curar enfermos."

116. Ibid.: "no el engrandecimiento personal ni el ridiculo privilegio de clase, sino ante todo el bien general, y consiguirán adquirir la posicion social que de derecho les corresponde, y de que tanto necesitan para labrar la ventura de la humanidad."

117. Martínez y Fernández, *Espejo del verdadero médico,* 13: "y en que por único galardon de los afanes solo se alcanza la ingratitud de los hombres, la continua agitacion, una posicion media, los desengaños de su impotencia y la melancólica satisfaccion de haber cumplido con su deber."

118. Nerea Aresti has commented on the pervasiveness of this ideal of the medical martyr: "The figure of the social physician was also contructed by way of a mythic component, approaching the image of the hero-martyr." See *Médicos, donjuanes y mujeres modernas,* 78–79.

119. Martínez y Fernández, *Espejo del verdadero médico,* 13: "¡feliz tú si la vocacion y el talento te guian para tan grande empresa! ¡desgraciado si el interés ó la ambicion es el móvil de tu preferencia! Si, amigos mios; si os sentís con ánimo resuelto á sufrir para saber poco, á arrostrar peligros para obtener desengaños, á vivir mártires para morir virtuosos, á gastar vuestro patrimonio para no reembolsar lo gastado, entonces penetrad en el templo; pero si os conoceis flojos, si no sabeis resistir las tentaciones, so no conoceis la virtud del heroismo, si no alcanzais el deber del sacrificio, retroced, no profaneis el templo de Esculapio."

120. On this phenomenon, see Nerea Aresti Esteban, "El ángel del hogar."

121. Martykánová and Núñez García, "Ciencia, patria y honor," 70–71.

122. See Arroyo, "Giving Birth to Science." For broad historical overviews of women's roles in providing healthcare throughout Europe, see Cabré and Ortiz-Gómez, eds., "Mujeres y salud: prácticas y saberes."

123. Bolufer i Peruga, "Cos femení, cos social," 532. On medical certification, see Albarracín Teulón, "La titulación médica en España durante el siglo XIX."

124. Martykánová and Núñez García, "Ciencia, patria y honor," 74: "La emulación era la dinámica clave: los hombres debían emular a los que habían logrado distinguirse por sus méritos superando todo tipo de obstáculos, y como premio por este esfuerzo serían emulados por otros."

125. Martínez, "Del influjo de lo físico en lo moral y vice-versa," 32–33.

3. On the Matter of Mind

1. Richardson, *British Romanticism and the Science of the Mind,* 6. Elizabeth Williams notes that, although Gall has sometime been portrayed as an opponent of Ideologues such as Cabanis, they in fact shared key assumptions, especially concerning the material bases of cognition (*The Physical and the Moral,* 106).

2. Reed, *From Soul to Mind,* 27.

3. Ibid., 25.

4. On Cousin's misconstrual of his philosophical forebears, see Reed, *From Soul to Mind,* 30–34. For a more detailed treatment of Cousin's influence, see chapters 4 and 5 in Goldstein, *Post-Revolutionary Self.*

5. Programas para las asignaturas de segunda ensenanza mandadas observar por S. M. en todos los institutos, seminarios y colegios del reino por Real Orden de 20 de setiembre de 1850, Madrid, Imprenta Nacional, 1850: "El profesor de la asignatura debe definir la psicologia manifestando detenidamente la existencia del alma, su distincion sustancial del cuerpo y de la materia, sus atributos de unidad, identidad y actividad y las facultades primarias e irreductibles del YO humano [sic], a saber: la sensibilidad, la inteligencia y la voluntad."

6. See, for example, Novella, *La ciencia del alma.* Novella quotes the above passage from the Spanish institutes of education (94n56) and discusses the influence of Cousin's eclecticism in Spain (93–99). He coins the phrase "militant spritualism" in "La política del yo."

7. Reed, *From Soul to Mind,* 44–45.

8. Bartolomé Alcalá y Pavon, "Fenómenos de la naturaleza," BH AP 4 leg. 1, doc. 20, 69: "Los Padres de la Yglesia que aparecieron despues, adoptando las ideas esparcidas sobre la es-piritualidad del alma, la consideraban como una emanacion inmediata de la divinidad y desde entonces se hizo opinion dominante de que este ser misterioso era una substancia inmaterial, eminentemente activa, inmortal, y que tenia la facultad de desear y pensar."

9. Ibid.: "Fué juzgado el hombre mirado como un ser escencial de la creacion y el unico capaz de discernir y juzgar en libertad. Los animales por el contrario se consideraban cual maquinas groseras sin facultades de distinguir y cuyos movimientos eran regulados por el inmutable y ciego destino. Tales son las ideas que cerca dos mil años han reynado en todas las naciones muy civilizados del mundo."

10. Ibid., 72: "En 1er lugar les diré a Vds. que soy un materialista puro; que considero imaginarios todos los entes espirituales que dicen los metafisicos que existen, que todas las religiones las considero como falsas y unicamente fundadas en la utilidad de interes de sus ministros; . . . que la religion cristiana la considero como una de las absurdas y en la que mas le deja conocer el espiritu lucrativo de sus ministros."

11. Ibid.: "Pero dejando estas consideraciones que son ajenas del asunto que nos ocupa; me voy á hablar esclusivamente de ese ser misterioso, espiritual, indivisible inmaterial que suponen existe en nuestro cuerpo."

12. Ibid., 72–74: "En 1er. lugar si se considera metafisicamente la existencia del alma veremos que es imaginaria y si no ¿Por donde podemos recibir un conocimiento de su existencia? ¿Porque ignoramos el mecanismo del cerebro en los actos intelectuales y esto será razon suficiente para admitir su existencia? No señores, pues entonces podiamos admitir con Bacon una alma sensitiva, por que se ignora el mecanismo de los nervios en los actos senstivos y en una palabra podriamos admitir en nuestro cuerpo tantos almas como funciones no fuesen desconocidas lo cual es un absurdo.

En 20. lugar yo preguntaria á los que admitan la existencia del alma ¿Como se puede admitir una cosa sin partes? ¿Como puede existir y ocupar un punto matematico? pues yo señores, no puedo comprehender que la existencia de un cuerpo sea compatible con la carencia de partes que pueda existir y no ocupar espacio, pues para mi decir esto, es decir que no existe. En vano se medirá que es un ente espiritual, que tiene propiedades distintas de los cuerpos materiales; pues yo preguntaré ¿Por donde, por que medios ó conductos se han podido analizar estas propiedades? La naturaleza nos ha dotado de ciertos sentidos externos é internos para que nos pongamos en relacion con los objetos que nos rodean, para que los estudiemos, para que estudiemos las cualidades buenas ó malas. en fin para que satisfagamos nuestras necesidades; . . . [S]olo podemos tener ideas de cosas materiales, solo de ellas podemos juzgar raciocinar con exactitud; . . . Y asi dejando aparte toda consideracion metafisica voy á examinar fisiologicamente la cuestion que es el modo que debo seguir para resolverla."

13. Ibid., 74–75: "el cerebro no es un organo unico, sino un compuesto de organos los cuales están encargados de ejecutar las diferentes facultades intelectuales y por consiguiente para que supone dos cosas, ó que el alma se divide en varias partes para precindir á los actos diversos de las diversas partes del encephalo ó que hay tantas almas diversas cuantos diversos organos cerebrales tenemos."

14. Ibid., 75.

15. Ibid., 79–80: "aunque haya manifestado que las religiones se fundan en un principio falso, tal es el conocimiento de la existencia del alma, estoy muy lejos de creer que semejantes instituciones sean inutiles, por el contrario ellas han sido las que han empezado la obra de la civilizacion en todos los pueblos, ellas solas enseñando á los hombres la esperanza de un mejor porvenir ó poseyendoles de un saludable terror podian superar al principio de esta carrera, los obstaculos que oponian al establecimiento del orden, los habitos todavia persistentes, aunque unas apagadas de la vida errante y la inclinacion casi irrestible del hombre al abuso de sus fuerzas. Los primeros legisladores aparecieron como inspirados por la divinidad, por todas partes hablaron á sus contemporaneos el mismo lenguaje é impusieron leyes morales sacadas del mismo origen."

16. Ibid.: "una base solida é inalterables, formar un conocimiento exacto y completo de la funcion mas noble y sublime de nuestra maquina."

17. Martínez y Fernández, *Médicos perseguidos por la Inquisición Española*, 51: "El materialismo es un sistema como otro cualquiera, y el hombre debe ser respetado, sea cualquiera su fe, si es sincera."

18. Martínez, "Tratado de fisiología #1," 2 (pagination mine).

19. See Martínez's notes to Oliva Sabuco's *Nueva filosofía*, 560–61

20. Martín Araguz, "Spanish Brain Science and Philosophy of Mind in the Time of Cervantes," 13.

21. The idea of a "Renaissance organicism" has been advanced by Barona Vilar in *Sobre medicina y filosofía natural en el Renacimiento*, 33–34. See also Martín Araguz, "Spanish Brain Science and Philosophy of Mind in the Time of Cervantes," 13. Mercedes Caridad García Gómez links Sabuco to the animism of Georg Ernst Stahl and the psychoanalisis of Freud in *La concepción de la naturaleza humana en la obra de Miguel Sabuco*, 153, 154. Alain Guy also links Sabuco to Stahl in "Miguel Sabuco, psicólogo de las pasiones," 121.

22. On Huarte's sources, see Read, *Juan Huarte de San Juan*, 47–59, and Guillermo Serés's introduction to the *Examen*, 70–107. On Sabuco, see Gianna Pomata's introduction to *The True Medicine*.

23. Martínez, "Del influjo de lo físico en lo moral y vice-versa," 6: "En efecto, señores, el influjo de lo moral en lo fisico estaba admitido generalmente en toda la antigüedad, y sobre esto no habia cuestion alguna, puesto que consideraban al cuerpo como el instrumento del alma, esta mandado y aquel obedeciendo, la una tirana y el otro esclavo."

24. Ibid.

25. Scholars have seen in Huarte a harbinger of contemporary theories on the modularity of mind. See García García, "Huarte de San Juan, un adelantado a la teoría modular de la mente."

26. Martínez, "Del influjo de lo físico en lo moral y vice-versa," 7–8: "La obra de este sabio compatricio, es una de aquellas que formó epoca no solo en la Medicina patria sino en la de Europa, y los hombres sabios de todas naciones, aprecian el merito de este español insigne." Martínez was not alone in connecting the work of Huarte with that of Gall. See, for example, Salvá, "Observaciones sobre la obra titulada *Examen de ingenios* por Juan Huarte, escritor a fines del siglo XVI."

27. Ibid., 8: "debe considerarse con tanto mayor merito cuanto que Huarte no podia aun espresar sus ideas de filosofia natural, como con muchos rodeos y no sin gracia refiere el mismo, respecto de ciertas cuestiones teologicas."

28. Balltondre Pla, "El conocimiento de sí y el gobierno de las pasiones en la obra de Sabuco," 108.

29. Barona, *Sobre medicina y filosofía natural*, 144–45.

30. Pomata, introduction to *The True Medicine*, 41–42.

31. Sabuco, *The True Medicine*, 101.

32. Ibid., 104.

33. Martínez, notes to Sabuco, *Nueva filosofía*, 511: "Si consideramos con calma y reflexion, que Alibert, hombre erudito á no dudarlo, escritor facil sin disputa alguna, ha compuesto su obra dosceintos años despues de nuestra Oliva, ciertamente nos pasmaremos de no encontrar mas adelantado al escritor francés que á la insigne doctriz española."

34. See Juan Mosácula, *Elementos de fisiología especial ó humana*, vol. 2 (Madrid, 1830). Félix Janer, *Gaceta Médica de Madrid*, November 29, 1834, 26; July 25, 1835, 8.

35. *Boletín del Instituto Médico Valenciano* 7 (October 1841): 4: "El hombre por su sistema moral es la perfeccion misma en el órden de la creacion."

36. Ibid., 7: "El creador delegó en el hombre una parte de su imperio sobre la tierra; formó una criatura noble, sublime, capaz de enlazar de algun modo la tierra con el cielo. Para tan alto destino fue preciso distinguir este noble término de la materia organizada con un rayo de sus facultades. Asi es que lo hizo libre, de otro modo no hubiera hecho otra cosa que modificar una porcion de materia al modo que la del bruto. Presentó á su vista la idea del bien y del mal, de lo justo é injusto, y le dijo: *eres libre.*"

37. Ibid., 8: "ese espíritu pensador depositario de la ciencia del bien y del mal. Esta, es, nuestra alma, esta, ese *yo* que discurre: el *yo* por quien registramos en un solo instante todas las partes de la tierra sin movernos lugar: ese *yo* que manda al cuerpo y este le obedece."

38. Martínez, notes to Sabuco, *Nueva filosofía*, 560: "es indudable que atenidos a los principios filosóficos y desarrollandolos con entera libertad, a mi me parece que se puede elegir un termino medio, a saber: seguir el eclecticismo ilustrado."

39. Ibid., 560: "En efecto, los unos quieriendo reducir al hombre á la condicion del animal, le rebajaban; pero es necesario hacerlos justicia, es mas lógico aun este sistema que el opuesto, que mientras ensalza al hombre espiritual hasta las nubes, colocándole en la categoria de los angeles."

40. Ibid., 558: "un no sé que . . . que nace y viene del Ser Supremo, una emanacion divina, una particilla especial en quien residen las facultades de la razon y del pensamiento, productos inmateriales como la causa que los produce, y que el cuerpo no puede modificar esencialmente sino de un modo accidental y accesorio. . . . [E]s independiente en su accion del organismo, y que es imperecedera é inmortal. . . . Los que defienden esta doctrina, miran al cuerpo como una pasividad que cede siempre que está bien organizado al alma."

41. Quoted by Novella, *La ciencia del alma*, 98: "La vida del alma es una vida que se conoce a sí misma, una fuerza autonómica o que se dirige por sí, y que tiene conciencia de su energía y de sus facultades; es una causa libre, es una *vita sui conscia, sui potens, sui motrix*. . . . Las fuerzas físicas son *autómatas;* la fuerza psíquica es *autócrata.*"

42. Martínez, notes to Sabuco, *Nueva filosofía*, 561: "El hombre se compone . . . de una fuerza que obra y ejecuta y se manifiesta mediante órganos corporales y materiales."

43. Ibid.: "Esta fuerza indemonstrable por sí misma por los sentidos y el raciocinio, sin embargo está alimentada y sostenida en nosotros por la conciencia íntima del yo." "[N]o podemos demonstrar las cualidades de que se encuentra adornada, y de consiguiente menos aun su naturaleza; de donde se deduce que solo conocemos su existencia por sus manifestaciones, y que estas manifestaciones esteriores, forman lo que debemos denominar sus leyes."

44. Ibid., 561–62: "Ahora bien, es indudable que, sea cual fuera su naturaleza, ella necesita de los órganos corporales como instrumentos á quienes manda y dirige en cierto modo, y que á medida que estos instrumentos son mas perfectos, aquella llena mejor su deseo y voluntad."

45. Ibid., 562: "Siendo indudable que el alma, como principio de actividad, modifica y determina la voluntad y los actos cuando el organismo obra armónicamente; tambien lo es que el cuerpo modifica las condiciones del alma por sensaciones esteriores que la determinan, que la fuerzan en cierto modo; de donde se concluye, que el cuerpo es tambien una actividad

en relacion con los objetos esteriores, que modifica al alma, y de consiguiente, el hombre es un doble compuesto de dos actividades, del cuerpo y del alma, de dos corrientes una interna centrífuga, que es el alma, y otra esterna centrípeta que es el cuerpo; que ambas se modifican mútuamente."

46. Ibid., 563: "He aqui, pues, el verdadero eclecticismo, el alma existiendo á la manera que queria Stahl, como facultad, como instrumentos obrando bajo aquella direccion."

47. De Ceglia, "Matter Is Not Enough," 505–6.

48. Plastina, "Oliva Sabuco de Nantes and Her Nueva Filosofia," 739. On the Aristotelian-Galenic paradigm, see Vidal, *The Sciences of the Soul*, 30–35.

49. Federspil and Sicolo, "The Nature of Life in the History of Medical and Philosophic Thinking," 339–40.

50. See, for example, Barthez, *Nouveaux éléments de la science de l'homme* 1: 19. It is indeed the case that many scholars have highlighted vitalist critiques of Stahl, but as Charles Wolfe shows, it is incorrect to characterize vitalism as "anti-Stahlian" ("The Animal Economy as Object and Program in Montpellier Vitalism," 544–45). A useful overview of the contentious debates over mechanism and vitalism during the period in question can be found in Hall, *Ideas of Life and Matter* 2.

51. Martínez, "Dissertation" 1840, 9: "¡Fanaticos mortales, dejad de inquirir las causas primitivas, esenciales, estudiad solo los efectos, observad, experimentad, interrogad con modestia a la naturaleza, y adelantereís en vuestras investigaciones! En efecto Señores ¿hemos adelantado nosotros mas la fisiologia, con la invencion del principio vital y los devaneos del Paracelso que con la observacion y practica de un Galeno y un Hipocrates? Ciertamente que no; antes bien hemos retardado los conocimientos y efectos debidos á alteraciones manifiestas en laorganizacion, los hemos atribuido a ese principio particular que muchas veces se le considera como inteligente, y otras no, que en suma desconocemos, no valiendo mas que manifestar nuestra insuficiencia, quedando tan convencidos con la palabra como si realmente supiesemos algo envolviendo en esa esplicacion la mas completa prueba de nuestra ignorancia, siendo de advertir que la palabra vital es á donde dirijimos los facultativos, aquello que no entendemos, como los fisicos á su atraccion, y los quimicos á su afinidad."

52. Williams, *The Physical and the Moral*, 47.

53. Martínez, "Disertacion," 9: "Bien conozco, Señores, que la vida es un efecto, que todo resultado supone causa y que para entendernos es preciso darle un nombre: para eso pues admito una causa que produce la vida (principio vital) y que por medio de la generacion transmite, da una propiedad general á todos los seres organicos."

54. Martínez, "Tratado de fisiología," #1, part 2, 5: "No viendonos posible seguir en esto otro sistema que el de los vitalistas, le adoptamos; porque es muy cierto que los fenomenos vitales no se pueden esplicar de otro modo, en razon de que cada fuerza fisica quimica no puede ser vital sin reunirse con otro elemento que la constituye en tal estado: por cuya razon quedan escluidas las teorias de los querian esplicar los fenomenos de la vida por solas leyes fisicas y quimicas, esclusivamente sino en asociacion con las leyes vitales."

55. Duffin, "Vitalism and Organicism in the Philosophy of R.-T.-H. Laennec," 536. On the difficulties involved in making neat distinctions between vitalism, mechanism, and materialism, see also Wolfe, "Forms of Materialist Embodiment." And Williams points out that even Léon Rostan, one of the chief proponents of nineteenth-century organicism, made use of vitalist concepts (*The Physical and the Moral*, 196).

56. Coleman, *Biology in the Nineteenth Century* (quoted by Duffin, "Vitalism and Organicism in the Philosophy of R.-T.-H. Laennec," 536).

57. López Piñero, "Las ciencias médicas en la España del siglo XIX," 218.

58. For an overview of this debate, see Ramos, "La polémica hipocrática en la medicina española del siglo XIX."

59. Mata and Martínez both served on a committee for the Spanish Medical Confederation in 1848. See *Gazeta Médica* III (January 30, 1848): 22. See Pedro Mata, *El Crisol* 14 (April 12, 1855): 4–7.

60. Fernández-Medina, *Life Embodied,* 216.

61. Ibid., 222.

62. López Piñero, "Las ciencias médicas en la España del siglo XIX," 222.

63. "Retratos médicos," *El Crisol* 7 (1855): 7.

64. Martínez y Fernández [Dr. Barlo-Vento], *La apología de los ciegos, ó la homeo-pato mania.*

65. Ibid., 6. Martínez cites the originator of homeopathy Samuel Hahnemann's own admission that his method was not based on clinical experiments: "en todas mis obras no aparece un esperimento clínico."

66. Laurent Cerise, *Exposé et examen critique du système phrénologique,* 251: "Violà un example, entre mille, que nos pourrions citer, de la conséquence matérialiste tireé logiquement d'une science fausse."

67. Olmo, "La posesión diabólica en el *Examen de ingenios para las sciencias.*" This analogy is also touched upon in Giglioni, "Between Galen and St Paul."

68. See Huarte, *Examen,* 110.

69. Ibid., 117: "[E]l ánima racional y el demonio se aprovechan para sus obras de las calidades materiales, y que con unas se ofenden, y con las contrarias reciben contento. Y que por esta razon apetecen estare en unos lugares, y huyen de otros sin ser corruptibles."

70. Cerise, *Exposé et examen critique du système phrénologique,* 251: "Huarte et ses contemporains, dans leur foi naïve, avaient accepté une science qui était loin de concorder avec elle; cette contradiction l'embarrassa souvent. Le docteur alla jusqu'à se demander si l'influence du diable qui cause les mauvaises inclinations peut agir sur l'homme autrement que par les mauvaises qualités corporelles dans lesquelles il aime à séjourner, et si l'action de Dieu peut produire les bonnes inclinations autrement que par les bonnes qualités corporelles dans les quelles il se complaît."

71. Martínez, introduction to Huarte, *Examen,* xxxi: "Creo, pues, que en menos palabras no se puede espresar mejor ni con mas sencillez el eclecticismo de la época actual."

72. Ibid.: "pero si atendemos á que Cerise es demasiado espiritualista, á que él mismo dice que el hombre es una actividad espiritual que manda á una pasividad carnal sin ayuda de la que nada puede hacer, facilmente se deducirá que estuvo algun tanto inconsecuente al atacar á Huarte, puesto que este no dice mas que el pensamiento de Cerise con diferentes palabras, pues repite muchas veces que el ánima para obrar necesita de órganos que sean sus instrumentos."

73. Cerise, *Exposé et examen critique du système phrénologique,* 39–40: "l'homme, est une activité qui se manifeste à l'aide d'instruments charnels. La source de cette activité ne saurait être dans ces instruments eux-mèmes qui ne se meuvent jamais spontanément, qui ont besoin d'être excités pour être mus, dont le caractère est une passivité absolue. Cette affirmation est

rigoureusement vraie, psychologiquement et physiologiquement. La phrénologie proclame au contraire que l'activité des organes est la source de toutes les déterminations et de toutes les opérations morales et intellectuelles de l'homme."

74. On this episode, see Eling and Finger, *Franz Joseph Gall.* The crusade against phrenology was not only political, but also physiological, as seen in the research of Jean-Pierre-Marie Flourens. See Harrington, *Medicine, Mind, and the Double Brain,* 9–11.

75. Mata y Fontanet, *Filosofía española,* x: "Las potencias del alma no pueden realizarse sin órganos, y toda actividad orgánica es funcional; por tanto, cae en el dominio y jurisdiccion de la fisiologia. Toda psicologia, que no sea funcional ó fisiológica, es completamente falsa."

76. Martínez, notes to *Examen,* 366: "no demos mucho crédito al espiritualismo, y habremos hecho mucho para no retrogradar á tiempos en que la medicina de las afecciones mentales estaba reducida á decir: '*las enfermedades del alma no nos corresponden: tratémoslas solo moralmente.*' . . . en fin, estudiemos mejor la fisiologia y adelantaremos mas en la patologia."

77. Martínez, notes to Sabuco, *Nueva filosofía,* 557: "atribuye cada funcion ó accion á un órgano respectivo, abstraccion hecha del dogma y de las creencias."

78. See Snell, *Portraits of the Insane,* chapter 7, "The Golden Age of Alienism."

79. Ackerknecht, *A Short History of Psychiatry,* 37–38. See also Goldstein, *Console and Classify,* 80–89.

80. Ildefonso Martínez y Fernández, "Enfermedades mentales," *El Crisol* 7 (1855): 6. "[E]l despotismo y los hábitos de la tiranía, ejercen gran influencia sobre los hombres, y producen muchas locuras, y especialmente suicidios, así es como al caer la libertad romana se vieron una multitud de suicidios y muchos locos y locas bajo los reinados de Tiberio, Calígula y demás emperadores que ejercieron la tiranía."

81. Ibid., 7: "los partidarios del régimen antiguo han hecho guerra eterna á las reformas."

82. Martínez y Fernández, "Asilos de locos, e historia critica de la locura," 10: "en España estamos muy atrasados en este ramo del saber, en comparacion á otras naciones mas felices."

83. Ibid., 18: "No son las revueltas politicas quien ha producido la mayor parte de las engenaciones mentales? Hablen, no las pasiones, hable la razon. Abreme los fastos de la historia del genero humano, y en ellos encontraremos ejemplos palpitantes de esta verdad."

84. Ibid., 19: "el fuego de la revolucion aun no estinto, el fanatismo religioso resucitado esa mezcla, esa confusion agitada de ideas y doctrinas opuestas y en lucha, son los elementos mas á proposito para la produccion de las enfermedades mentales."

85. Ibid., 38–39: "habiendo muy pocos en España que hayan dedicado al dificil estudio del hombre como una dualidad compuesta de cuerpo y alma, que a la vez aparece como animal y otras como racional ó humanal propiamente dicho; siendo sobradamente cierto que no se han tratado de hermanar entre nosotros los principios de la escuela de Platon, Kant, Leibnitz, Malebranche, Descartes, y filosofos espiritualistas con los de Lock, Condillac, Destutt de Tracy, Cabanis, y Broussais ó sea la escuela organista no se puede sacar mucho partido de los estudios medicos que hemos aprendido en las escuelas."

86. On Nieto, see Riera, "Matias Nieto y Serrano (1813–1902) y la medicina romántica."

87. Nieto y Serrano, "Identidad del sueño y de la locura," *El Siglo Médico* 82 (July 29, 1855): 233: "No se busque relacion necesaria de causalidad entre los diversos órdenes de fenómenos que ofrece el organismo humano, entre la estructura del cerebro, por ejemplo, y los actos intelectuales y afectivos."

88. Ibid.: "En resúmen, se trata de saber si un poco de dureza ó de blandura, de rubicundez ó de palidez, si algo mas ó menos de sangre en el cerebro, si alguna otra por fin de las lesiones visibles y tangibles que se encuentran en el cadáver, produce el trastorno de las facultades del alma que se llama locura; ó si un espiritu, una cosa inmaterial que debe admitirse como causa de la vida y de la razon independientemente de los órganos, es el que se altera por si, dando consecutivamente lugar á las lesiones materiales que se encuentran algunas veces en los sugetos afectados."

89. Sabuco, *Nueva filosofía*, 483: "La causa y oficina de los humores de toda enfermedad es el cerebro; alli están las pasiones, afectos, y movimientos del ánima."

90. Sabuco, *New Philosophy of Human Nature*, ed. Waithe, Colomer Vintró, and Zorita, 254–55.

91. Martínez, notes to Huarte, *Examen*, 355: "Pero no solo queria Huarte que se le dijere donde residian los vicios y virtudes, sino que deseaba le indicasen la terapéutica de las pasiones, el modo de curarlas; pues acaso con su gran injenio habia alcanzado el grave y dificil estudio de las perturbaciones morales en que han adelantado tanto en estos últimos tiempos Pinel y Esquirol."

92. Ibid., 364.

93. Ibid., 365–66: "Por lo demas solo colocamos esto como hipótesis, mientras que un estudio mas profundo y filosófico no venga á con vencernos de lo contrario ó de sus pruebas, y no nos cansaremos de repetir que el estudio dificilísimo de las enfermedades mentales aun no ha comenzado; puede decirse que es empírico y no filosófico; porque la fisiologia no ha hecho aun bastante acerca del estudio moral y físico del hombre."

94. Ibid., 363.

95. Martínez, notes to Sabuco, *Nueva filosofía*, 574: "La locura es una afeccion cerebral, ordinariamente crónica, sin fiebre, caracterizada por desórdenes de la sensibilidad, de la inteligencia y de la voluntad."

96. Ibid., 507: "fuera de todo monopolio orgánico esclusivo."

97. Novella, "La política del yo," 464.

98. García Caballero, *De la libertad moral en sus relaciones con los delitos*, 7: "Es el hombre á lo que se ve, un compuesto de dos sustancias: inmaterial, espiritual, inteligente, activa, sensible, con voluntad y libertad moral la una, llamada ordinariamente, alma, espíritu: la otra, material por naturaleza, incapaz de pensamiento y de sentimientos llamada cuerpo, que es la materia organizada, resultado de partículas divisibles con movimiento y vida prestados por una potencia inmaterial, y sugeta á alteraciones, cambios, leyes distintas, destrucción y muerte."

99. Ibid., 8: "Los mas aventajados filólosofos que creen en la omnipotencia cerebral, escluyendo á fortiori la existencia del alma, del espíritu humano como juez regulador de todo,centro del pensamiento y de los sentimientos que ennoblecen y divinizan al hombre, haciendo al cerebro el dictador de las acciones que llamamos buenas y malas, y de consiguiente al hombre, un servil y abyecto dependiente de su organización. . . . fijan ;que el alma no existe: que la percepción, las ideas, el juicio, memoria, voluntad y las afecciones, son inmediato resultado de la acción cerebral, ó mejor, modos de escitacion del sistema nervioso; siendo las virtudes y vicios la consecuencia de la lucha del órgano encefálico y las principales visceras, cuyas variadas modificaciones percibidas por el sensorio forman nuestras pasiones. ¡Qué sensibles errores!. . . ¡qué filosofismo tan grosero! hacer depender la nobleza humana, la razón, de la materia! Gran

número de pruebas se me agolpan en contra de esta filosofía de los Hobbe, Espinosa, y sus discípulos Heltvetius, Lamettrie, y los Gall, Broussais, etc."

100. "De la libertad moral en sus relaciones con los delitos," *El Siglo Médico* 54 (January 14, 1855).

101. Martínez y Fernández, "O petulancia, osadia," *El Crisol* 6 (1855): 10: "el Sr. Caballero conoce *poco, poquisimo,* la fisiologia intelectual, la anatomía-patalógica cerebral; es decir, niega el cuerpo no solo el pensamiento, sino lo que es mas, el *sentimiento*. . . . qué idea tendrá de las locuras, cómo se reirá el pobre fisiólogo Mangendi [*sic*] que estableció "que el cerebro es el órgano material del pensamiento." Pobres gentes, pobre Cabanis, infeliz Broussais, insensato Huarte. . . . y todo esto ¿para qué? para deducir de una mentira fisiológica una verdad sociológica, la inmortalidad del alma. . . . dejemos es mitad á la teologia y á la Iglesia."

102. Ibid., 10–11: ¿me hace V. el favor de darme un alma humana parlante y pensadora separada del cerebro y de la cabeza del hombre?" "y esa quisicosa es el *alma,* porque sin ella no habria *yo,* y sin yo habria . . . confusion y barullo y anarquia."

103. Ibid., 11: "y sobre todo estudie V. el cerebro v sus cruzamientos y sus confluentes, y advertirá donde esta el *yo* del sistema nervioso general."

104. Ibid.: "¡Estranjeros médico-legistas, fisiólogos y anatómicos, no nos juzgeis en patologia mental por la memoria que analizamos! ¡Quiera el cielo *que no haya* pasado el Pirineo, y no tengamos que sufrir las consecuencias de la *osadia* de ciertos escritores cis-pirenáicos! No, no, fisiólogos y médicos distinguidos; la patologia mental está mas adelantada entre nosotros de lo que aparece en la memoria que acabamos de analizar, y sabed que hay profesores modestos que tienen conocimientos mas sólidos sobre enfermedades mentales."

105. Martínez y Fernández, "Enfermedades mentales," *El Crisol* 7 (1855): 3: "La locura es una enfermedad material ó espiritual, ó mejor dicho, las afecciones mentales son enfermedades orgánicas ó son del alma?"

106. Ibid., 3–4: "la actividad del alma depende de la integridad de la estructura anatómica y de la composicion quimica del cerebro."

107. Ibid., 4: "el médico solo tiene que ocuparse de todas las aberraciones de las facultades intelectuales, tan solo del cambio material que obliga al alma á acciones morbosas, ó que le impide obrar; por consecuencia, en los casos de alteraciones orgánicas no se puede suponer una enfermedad innata del alma sin defecto primordial del principio moral, pues un cambio repentino del estado del cerebro hiere instantáneamente de enfermedad las manifestaciones del alma."

108. Ibid.: "las manias son un género de enfermedades que no se diferencian enteramente de las demás afecciones del cerebro, pues son consecuencia muy frecuente de ellas las apoplegias, epilepsias, y paralisis."

109. Ibid., 5: "establecen indudablemente que todas las facultades del hombre son adherentes a su encéfalo, que nacen, crecen, se alteran, se disminuyen, se aumentan destruyen con este instrumento material."

110. Ibid., 6: "En conclusion, nosotros pensamos con Frank, Huarte, Broussais, Cabanis y la mayor parte de los autores, que la locura es una enfermedad material nerviosa, agena de ninguna modification esencial del alma, porque admitir enfermedades de un principio espiritual, idéntico en todos los individuos, lo creemos absurdo, antimoral e irreligioso."

111. Ibid.: "pensamos con los organicistas, si bien aun no han podido descubrirse alter-

aciones constantes; pero esperamos que con el tiempo lleguen á distinguirse estas enfermedades con caracteres orgánicos, como lo son hoy dia la apoplegia, la paralisis, la epilepsia."

112. García Caballero, *De la libertad moral en sus relaciones con los delitos,* 24: "Así cumplirá
con su mision el hombre en la tierra; ser para la sociedad; que si impone á los asociados
deberes recíprocos para la comun felicidad, tambien ofrece en cambio seguridad y garantías
contra las pretensiones y atropellos del mas fuerte , estableciendo asi la paz y la armonía entre
los pueblos , y la dicha y bien-estar de cada uno de los miembros que componen un mismo
cuerpo político."

113. Ibid., 22: "El hombre, ser el mas admirable de la creación, es un compuesto de dos sustancias distintas, *alma, cuerpo.* Cada uno de estos elementos de su ser, tiene atributos y propiedades esenciales, parte dependientes parte independientes que le someten á leyes distintas, y
como á existencias distintas: el cuerpo, á las leyes trazadas por el Criador, á la materia; el alma,
á las que plació dar á los espíritus el soberano Hacedor de quien procede á quien vuelve."

114. Ibid.: "el fatalismo atroz y desanimador del *acto forzoso* á que los materialistas conde-
nan á la humanidad."

115. See Lakoff and Johnson, *Metaphors We Live By.*

116. See, for example Zavadil, "Anatomy of the Body Politic," 51–58. See also Musolff,
"Political Metaphor and Bodies Politic."

117. On these processes, see Trim, *Metaphor and the Historical Evolution of Conceptual
Mapping.*

118. Martínez, "Tratado de fisiología #2," 6v.

119. Like Martínez, Amich was a fierce critic of *moderado* liberalism, as evidenced by his
bitter denuciation of the Moderate Party, whose "Machiavellian plans" contributed to the
suppression of the Barcelona uprising of 1842–43 (Amich, *Acontecimientos políticos,* 8).

120. Juan Amich, "La frenología no es utopia, no se opone á la libertad del alma, es útil á la
medicina," *El Porvenir Médico* 36 (September 30, 1853): 147.

121. Ibid.: "Dudamos primero de la frenología, y aun pretendimos combatirla; pero la
estudiamos y al momento fuimos partidario de su doctrina."

122. Ibid.: "El cerebro está dividido en diferentes partes ú órganos, destinados á funciones
especiales, sujetos á un *centro comun indivisible,* el alma."

123. Ibid.: "es el alma el soberano el entendimiento; colocado en su solio convoca á sus
órganos inmediatos, quienes mancomunadamente funcionan, trasladando se es preciso sus
órdenes á los demas, para que obedezcan el legislativo poder."

124. Juan Amich, "La medicina y la política," *El Porvenir Médico* 105 (September 15, 1854):
204: "En el estudio del hombre hallamos leyes constantes que aprender leyes dictadas por la
naturaleza y no fruto de la inteligencia humana."

125. Ibid.: "No hay órgano que en sus funciones pueda llamarse soberano; la soberania está
en el todo y no en la parte; cada sistema de órganos se rige por leyes especiales, nuestra economia puede compararse á una porcion de pueblos confederados que se ausilian reciprocamente
y de esta armonia resulta la felicidad y órden social como de aquella la salud y la vida. Desde
el momento en que algun órgano pretende hacerse superior, su pletora dá por resultado la
enfermedad, el enflaquecimiento de los demas sistemas de órganos, como sucede á los pueblos
en que el predominio de uno, ó algunos pocos constituye la esclavitud de los mas; pero en la
naturaleza del hombre se efectuan revoluciones completas, triunfa el todo ó muere el todo con

la parte; hay unidad, porque no existe intersticio ni tegido alguno que no rechaze con energia la parte morbitica; pueden sucumbir, es cierto, pero nadie les quita la gloria de haber resistido hasta acabar por último con el tirano."

126. Ibid.: "Mira con igual celo al microscópico filete nervioso que á la masa encefalica en cuyo centro se efectuan los tan maravillosos fenómenos de la inteligencia. A propósito de estos fenómenos ¿qué deducimos de su estudio? la imposibilidad de coartar su libertad absoluta, porque el autor de la naturaleza le ha impuesto la ley de ejercerla completamente. En esa masa hallamos tambien su constitucion federativa, obrando cada circulo en entera independencia, siendo los demás meros ausiliares; se forma un juicio, acude en su ausilio la memoria, la comparacion, la causalidad, la circumspeccion etc., quiere ejecer un acto benévolo ó bien al contrario, el circulo activo si quiere, consulta á los demás y resuelve siempre con entera libertad; he aqui porque proclamamos los mas la libertad del pensamiento y hasta de la conciencia, la que como las demás libertades no puede tener límites."

127. Ibid.: "ese orgullo y esa riqueza de los magnates al lado de esas chozas en que el hambre es la única soberana"; "no es justo haya una distancia tan inmensa entre los hombres como la que existe entre la opulencia y la miseria."

128. Ibid.: "En nuestra economia esperimentamos que en estado normal, todos los órganos ejercen sus respectivas funciones y existe la asimilacion en todos ellos ¿por qué pues todas las clases de la sociedad no deben ser protejidas para poder satisfacer sus necesidades?"

129. Ibid.: "sus opiniones deben de estar enlazadas á los principios liberales, porque tenemos por base la tolerancia, la amabilidad, la filantropia, procurando el alivio con iqual esmero en las dolencias del absolutista como en las del republicano; del católico, como del protestante ó mahometano; cada uno marche :do quiera; vaya al cielo por donde le de la gana."

130. Ibid.

131. Amich, "La medicina y la política: Estudio comparativo de los poderes del estado y órden administrativo con la organizacion del hombre," *El Porvenir Médico* 107 (September 25, 1854): 211–12.

132. Ibid.: "esa misma democracia degeneraria en una oligarquia ó bien en una dictadura, se el jefe elegido pudiera disponer de los intereses y destinos del pais."

133. Ibid.: "Disputemos pues este importante punto y veamos si en la organizacion del hombre hallamos leyes que aprender."

134. Cobb, "A Brief History of Wires in the Brain." For a more extensive treatment of brain metaphors in the nineteenth century see, by the same author, *The Idea of the Brain,* chapter 4.

135. Amich, "La medicina y la política: Estudio comparativo de los poderes del estado y órden administrativo con la organizacion del hombre," 211–12: "Ha organizado el sistema de funciones y por medio de los filites nerviosos como verdadera telegrafia humana las ha puesto en armonia con la inteligencia, que la consideramos como el poder ejecutivo."

136. Ibid., 212: "El poder legislativo pertenece á la naturaleza, y su constitucion la forman todos los elementos y en consecuencia el mismo hombre. El ejecutivo colocado en su parte superior, tal es la intelegencia, con los cordones nerviosos que la ponen en relacion consigo mismo y con el esterior. El órden administrativo que lo constituyen dos grandes funcionarios, el aparato digetivo con sus vasos linfáticos y venosos que llevan los liquidos destinados á la nutricion, el centro del aparato circulato-rio; y este centro que recibe la sancion del poder

legislativo encarandose luego de que por medio de los conductos arteriales, se efectue la asimilacion en toda nuestra economia, es decir, el poder ejecutivo limitado y la administracion, parte del legislativo."

137. Ibid.: "Consideremos á el pueblo soberano: representada su soberania por un número de individuos elegidos del pueblo y por el pueblo con la facultad de legislar, ordenar la administracion y nombrar los funcionarios públicos incluso el poder ejecutivo." "[S]olo asi comprendemos la armonia, la salud y la vida de los pueblos, de lo contrario la inmoralidad y en consecuencia la enfermedad y la muerte del pais."

138. Ibid.: "Quitemos las garras al leeon y le perderemos el temor. Las garras del poder ejecutivo consisten en esa facultad que se le concede de disponer casi de un modo absoluto de los bienes de la patria y de sus administrativos, resultando de ahí que su insaciable hidrópica sed de oro puede dar por resultado la miseria de todo el pueblo, y con el mismo oro retribuir con prodigalidad á sus empleados, convertiendoles en fieles servidores de su señor."

139. Ibid.: "Apliquemos pues tambien el pronto remedio antes de que contamine el mal á los demas funcionarios."

140. See, for example, "Body Politic: Definition, History, & Facts," *Encyclopedia Britannica*, www.britannica.com/topic/body-politic (accessed May 20, 2022).

141. Elmer, *The Miraculous Conformist*, 8.

4. Medical Martyrs

1. *Boletín del Instituto Médico Valenciano* 11 (February 1842): 7: "Uno de los principales objetos que debe proponerse el que se dedica á una ciencia, es formar una idea exacta de su estado y adelantos por la comparacion de sus varias épocas y desarrollo progresivo de sus proposiciones ó verdades. Desgraciadamente para nosotros la medicina, si bien es la que necesita mas este estudio especial para comprender con exactitud sus diferentes revoluciones y sistemas, es tambien la que mas carece de obras filosóficas que permitan á un profesor el conocer por principios la historia de su arte."

2. Bujosa Homar, *Filosofía e historiografía médica en España*, 63–65.

3. Martínez y Fernández, "Las historias de la medicina de Chinchilla y Morejón," 380–82.

4. In one of the most famous plagiarism scandals in nineteenth-century Spanish letters, Chinchilla was accused of borrowing materials from Morejon's work. See Aguirre Marco, "Hernández Morejón, Anastasio Chinchilla y la historia de la medicina española," 133–41.

5. Ibid., 145–46.

6. Martínez y Fernández, "Las Historias de La Medicina de Chinchilla y Morejón," 380: "el señor Chinchilla se deja llevar de su entusiasmo patrio."

7. Dufour, "Juan Antonio Llorente: de corifeo del afrancesamiento a mártir del liberalismo," 48.

8. See Haliczer, "Inquisition Myth and Inquisition History."

9. Martínez y Fernández, *Médicos perseguidos por la Inquisición española*, 3: "No vamos ¡oh españoles! a recordar escenas sangrientas por gusto, vamos si á dar á conocer hechos poco conocidos, pero ciertos: atended y escarmentad, no en brazos de los mártires, sino en odio á los verdugos y tiranos del pensamiento. El pensamiento español perseguido por la Inquisición

pudiera llenar muchos tomos, pero la institución de los reyes católicos, analizada médicamente, puede dar origen a grandes comentarios."

10. Ibid., 34: "los fundadores de la mayor parte de religiones han sido, y probablemente serán, esclusivos, partidarios de su autoridad, celosos de sus perogativas, y solo Jesucristo, en cuanto hombre, fué lo contrario, porque era verdaderamente Dios y hombre á un mismo tiempo, y su mansedumbre, y su humildad, y su caridad, y su benevolencia, ni han sido imitadas sino en muy pequeña escala, ni por los cristianos *romanos*, ni por los *reformistas*."

11. Ibid.: "No es, pues, estraño que los *inquisidores*, que los *reformistas* sacrifiquen al hombre que piensa, que quiere, que cree diferentemente a lo que ellos quieren, piensan y creen; porque este es el efecto de toda escuela, de toda doctrina, de toda autoridad ordenada, pues unicamente la libertad individual constituida en toda su estension, esto es, fundada en la inviolabilidad de la conciencia humana, es la que puede respetar cualquier idea individual, por estravagante, por exagerada, por contraria que sea al sentido comun; de donde se concluye, que desde el momento que se crea un orden privilegiado, una escuela, una iglesia autorizada, desde aquel momento nace la persecution, la coaccion moral, los atractivos, y los castigos para los disidentes, para los incredulos, para los que piensan diferentemente del cuerpo oficial, legalizado y consentido; esto sucede lo mismo en España que en Francia, en Alemania como en Suiza, y de aqui el que, lo mismo los *catolicos romanos* que los *reformistas anglicanos*, llevan en si, aun en medio de la tolerancia, el germen de autoridad de secta, que unido a la envidia de las grandes cualidades de Servet, produjeron su inevitable ruina."

12. Ibid., 84: "víctimas ilustres y dignas, porque lo fueron de su ciencia." "De todas las ciencias no hay una que toque tan de cerca á la solucion del principio de libertad como la anatomía y fisiología . . . La filosofía del porvenir será una fisiología perfeccionada." Like Martínez, Esquiros was a writer of martyrologies. In 1840 he published *l'evangile du peuple*, which cast Christ as a social reformer, and in 1851 he published *Histoire des martyrs de la liberté*, which cast social reformers as Christlike martyrs.

13. Martínez y Fernández, *Médicos perseguidos por la Inquisición española*, 94: "¡Salud, oh grandes médicos perseguidos por la inquisicion: sí, salud, ilustres mártires; vosotros sufristeis los unos la encarcelacion, los otros el San Benito, algunos el destierro, otros la hoguera, pero vuestros comprofesores en la ciencia han hecho arrancar á vuestros tiranos infinitas víctimas, y les han dado en vez de verdugos caritativos hermanos!"

14. Torrecilla, *España al revés*, 39–40: "El rechazo de la España oficial les lleva a identificarse con todos aquellos grupos que habian sido víctimas del autoritarismo y la intolerancia de sus dirigentes. . . . Excluidos de la identidad española por los que pretendian monopolizar en exclusiva el espacio nacional, como si fueran sus unicos y legítimos propietarios, proponen a su vez que la España mas auténtica era precisamente la de aquellos grupos que habian sido amputados del tronco común por defender sus creencias, la de los perseguidos, exiliados y ajusticia-dos en nombre de una verdad que no era la suya. Ademas, al identificarse con esos grupos, proyectan sobre ellos sus ideas, como si el ser víctimas de una misma intolerancia estab-leciera entre ellos una comunidad de pensamiento."

15. Martínez y Fernández, "Juan Huarte," 89: "En tan desgraciada época y cuando el poder inquisitorial estaba mas en fuerza, es cuando Huarte se lanza á escribir un Exámen de Ingénios y á dedicar un articulo exclusivamente para representar las cualidades de que debiera estar dotado un Rey, sin dejar de manifestar las muchas condiciones que exigian los jurisperi-

tos, los sacerdotes, los medicos y todas las clases sociales, atacando preocupaciones arraigadas, tachando abusos y penet-rando una senda aun desconocida hasta él, teniendo que compaginar por el esfuerzo de su ingenio muchas cosas que si hubiera escrito en época mas bonancible no se hubiera curado ni aun de justificarlas."

16. The seminal text on the topic is Anderson, *Imagined Communities*.

17. Gracia Guillén, "Judaism, Medicine, and the Inquisitorial Mind in Sixteenth-Century Spain," 375. On the role of physicians in the Inquisition, see also Pardo-Tomás and Martínez Vidal, "Victims and Experts: Medical Practitioners and the Spanish Inquisition." For a comparative perspective, see Ruggiero, "The Cooperation of Physicians and the State in the Control of Violence in Renaissance Venice." See also Keitt, "The Miraculous Body of Evidence."

18. Ibid., 384–85.

19. Ibid., 388.

20. Ibid., 389. See also Sumillera, "Political Medicine in Early Modern Spain."

21. Sabuco, *Nueva filosofía*, 450.

22. Ibid., 480–81: "pues el médico es el ministro de las grandezas y secretos que Dios y su causa segunda la naturaleza criaron." "Y asi suplico á los sábios y cristianos médicos juzguen este negocio con equidad y justicia, pues les hacemos bien, y no mal, quitando lo errado y nocivo, y dándoles lo acertado y útil para ellos y para las repúblicas."

23. Ibid., 470: "Pues no es menor yerro el que el vulgo hace cada dia en los casamientos, no mirando mas de la hacienda y riqueza, olvidando lo principal que es la perfeccion de naturaleza en la persona, como se ve cada dia, y es cosa notoria ver las faltas de los padres en los hijos."

24. Ibid., 473n: "Todo este bellisimo trozo y los siguientes estan conformes con las ideas del celebre Huarte."

25. Ibid., 475: "Buscas y examinas un caballo para padre por tener buenos caballos, y ¿no examinarás al hombre que ha de ser padre de tus nietos y descendientes, para tener buenos nietos y decendientes, hombres habiles y no bestias?"

26. See Jorge Enríquez, *Retrato del perfecto médico*, 145.

27. Ibid., 147; quoted by Gracia Guillén, "Judaism, Medicine, and the Inquisitorial Mind in Sixteenth-Century Spain," 389–90: "Y mas que el Medico que fuere de rostro hermoso, no podra dexar de tener buena habilidad, è ingenio, y otras partes, que son necessarias para vno ser perfecto Medico, que regla es de philosophia que las costumbres del alma siguen el temple y complexion de cuerpo, como Galeno lo muestra en vn libro."

28. Ibid., 50; see Gracia Guillén, "Judaism, Medicine, and the Inquisitorial Mind in Sixteenth-Century Spain," 393.

29. Ibid., 31; quoted by Gracia Guillén, "Judaism, Medicine, and the Inquisitorial Mind in Sixteenth-Century Spain," 393: "[E]stavan obligados a hazer los Reyes y principes passados para auer de gouernar el mundo: y porque no lo haran los Medicos para regir el cuerpo del hombre que se llama mundo pequeño."

30. Gracia Guillén, "Judaism, Medicine, and the Inquisitorial Mind in Sixteenth-Century Spain," 382.

31. Ibid., 384.

32. Ibid., 391.

33. Ibid.

34. See Arrizabalaga and Giordano, "Cristianismo Paulino."

35. Williams, *The Physical and the Moral,* 207.

36. Cohen, *The French Encounter with Africans,* 233.

37. Varela de Montes et al., *Ensayo de antropología,* xiv–xv: "esa relacion íntima que existe entre lo físico y lo intelectual del Hombre."

38. Ibid., xv: "Si no se hubiera tomado en cuenta la organizacion para esplicar la moral y el entendimiento, yo me hubiera limitado al Hombre fisiológico; pero cuando veo y cuando oigo que todo es producto del organismo, yo debo hacerme cargo de estas cuestiones, ó para apoyarlas como fisiológicas, ó para rechazarlas ó situarlas en su verdadero terreno. Es esto tanto mas necesario y urgente, cuanto mas se ven prodigadas y con profusion repartidas entre la juventud las obras que *materializan* al Hombre, formando de sus deberes una institucion arbitraria."

39. Ibid., xv–xvi.

40. Ibid., 159, 160: "Comparadas las facultades intelectuales en las diversas razas, no pueden formarse del género humano familias distintas." "Es inútil la clasificacion de la especie humana, por que no trae ventaja alguna y nos induce á error.

41. Ibid., 159, 160: "Comparadas las facultades intelectuales en las diversas razas, no pueden formarse del género humano familias distintas." "El género humano forma una gran nacion compuesta de 934 millones de individuos."

42. Martinez, notes to Huarte, *Examen,* 392.

43. Ibid., 397: "Al decir el Sr. Varela que todos tienen unos mismos elementos intelectuales, generalizó demasiado."

44. Ibid., 392–93. "[L]os dos puntos mas dificiles que hay que resolver en fisiología á saber." "1a. El género humano depende de distintos troncos, con distintos caracteres." "2a. El género humano es único . . . , y la diferencia que existe en las variedades de la organizacion, son dependientes de circunstancias accidentales, que el clima, el tiempo, los hábitos."

45. Ibid., 393: "Cualquiera que sea nuestra opinion acerca de tan graves cuestiones, pasaremos á analizarlas con todo el criterio debido para despues deducir lo que debemos, acerca de las ideas de nuestro Huarte."

46. Cabanis, *On the Relations between the Physical and Moral Aspects of Man,* 450.

47. Huarte, *Examen,* 36: "Las costumbres del ánimo, siguen el temperamento del cuerpo donde está, y que por razon del calor, frialdad, humedad y sequedad de la region que habitan los hombres y de los manjares que comen, y de las aguas que beben, y del aire que respiran, unos son necios y otros sabios."

48. Martinez, notes to Huarte, *Examen,* 36n: "Esto prueba como Huarte se adelantó á Cabanis y Broussais, en la consideracion del hombre físico sobre el hombre moral."

49. Huarte, *Examen,* 194–95.

50. Ibid., 198.

51. Ibid., 201.

52. Ibid., 201: "Y de la manera que los negros comunican en España el color á sus descendientes por la simiente sin estar en Etiopia, asi el pueblo de Israel viniendo tambien á ella, puede comunicar á sus descendientes la agudeza de ingenio, sin estar en Egipto ni comer del maná, porque ser necio ó sabio, tambien es accidente del hombre como ser blanco ó negro." It is un-

clear where Huarte derived this story, since there is no reference to these Ethiopian emigrees in the Old Testament.

53. Ibid., 193.

54. Arrizabalaga and Giordano, "Cristianismo Paulino," 368.

55. See Cohen, *The French Encounter with Africans,* 211.

56. Varela de Montes et al., *Ensayo de antropología,* 170: "La influencia de los climas se estiende á obrar sobre el Hombre físico y sobre sus disposiciones á corresponder á las influencias intelectuales, pero no tiene un poder como se creyó con demasiada generalidad."

57. Ibid., 159: "Comparadas las facultades intelectuales en las diversas razas, no pueden formarse del genero humano familias distintas."

58. Ibid., 149: "Comparando Buffon la estructura cerebral del orango y de su voz con las del Hombre, y al hallarlas enteramente iguales, no pudo menos de concluir que la materia sola, aunque perfectamente organizada, no podia producir el pensamiento, . . . á no estar animada por un principio superior."

59. Martinez, notes to Huarte, *Examen,* 400.

60. Ibid.

61. Ibid., 401–2: "En efecto, ó las diferencias de las razas dependen de los climas ó no; si lo primero, no cabe la menor duda que la diferencia de organizacion depende de los climas, y en este caso, siendo la inteligencia hija de la organizacion, (pues llevamos probado que la alma en todos es igual; sino seria suponer una impiedad y una cosa imposible) facilmente se deduce que segun varie la organizacion, asi varía la inteligencia."

62. Ibid., 402: "no dependen de los climas y alimentacion dependerán de la conformacion orgánica primitiva, y por consecuencia de las razas que rechaza el Sr. Varela ó del alma, principio inmaterial del que nada sabemos y del que únicamente podemos suponer la ecsistencia, pero sin juzgar de su actividad."

63. Ibid.: "por mas que Bufon diga otra cosa, es lo cierto que nadie duda de la existencia de su cuerpo y de atribuir propiedades, mas facil era atribuir como propiedad del cuerpo al alma, que no al cuerpo como propiedad de una cosa que la ciencia no demuestra, que la razon apenas alcanza , y que el sentimiento solo acoge; pero de cuya cosa ninguna muestra tenemos."

64. Ibid., 402–3: "Hemos, pues, probado en mi entender cuanto era necesario; hemos discutido con franqueza y sin miedo ninguno nuestras opiniones, concluiré con manifestar, que admitiendo Huarte la disposicion innata, orgánica, y admitiendo al mismo tiempo que á igualdad de circunstancias los hombres eran mas despejados segun los favoreciesen los climas."

65. Ibid., 403: "la primera disposicion es la orgánica, la segunda el clima y demas que le rodean al hombre."

66. Varela de Montes et al., *Ensayo de antropología,* 132–33: "Los pueblos del Cáucaso . . . se consideran hoy dia como los mas hermosos Hombres de la tierra"; "aparece una distancia inmensa entre el caucasiano y el negro."

67. Martinez, notes to Huarte, *Examen,* 403: "No creemos que se nos tache de materialistas por personas sobradamente scrupulosas, pero por si sucediese, advertimos de ahora para entonces, que somos religiosos sin hipocresia, y que defendemos nuestras opiniones filosóficos con el raciocinio, sin pensar para nada en las que en el medio de hallar la verdad que buscamos con anhelo y que deseamos encontrar; si bien creemos que esta no se encuentra en un eclec-

ticismo que no tiene de esto mas que el nombre, y cuyo verdadero terreno es el espiritualismo disfrazado."

68. Ibid., 201n1: "Hé aqui una idea que un autor moderno de mucho mérito reproduce en nuestros dias, para espresar la constancia de los instintos en las diferentes especies y familias de animales; fundándose que es un caracter que se transmite por la generacion, no solo organi- camente sino las disposiciones, y aun añade que la educabilidad; de modo que un caballo docil y bien enseñado, producirá otro docil y bien enseñado tambien, o con gran disposicion para educarse y asi de las de mas especies; lo que sirve de fundamento al buscar un ser perfecto de la especie para la reproduccion."

69. Huarte, *Examen*, 256: "como los padres han de engendrar los hijos sabios." "[S]i esto pudiésemos remediar con arte, habriamos hecho á la republica el mayor beneficio que se le podria hacer." "Positive eugenics" meaning here the goal of encouraging those with desired traits to reproduce, as opposed to a negative eugenics that seeks to keep those with undersired traits from reproducing.

70. Ibid., 322: "de padres sabios salen hijos muy necios, y de padres necios hijos muy avisados."

71. Ibid., 309, 334.

72. Martinez, notes to Huarte, *Examen*, 407–8: "En efecto, esta combinacion entre temperamentos diferentes es muy buen precepto, y si fuese posible ponerle en práctica . . . se conseguiria la mejora de la especie humana."

73. *Boletín de medicina, cirugía, y farmacía* 2 (1847): 352: "ciertos individuos atacados de enfermedades terribles a la sociedad. Cierto que mucho se tendría adelantado para la mejora de la especie humana."

74. Ibid., 344.

75. Martinez, notes to Huarte, *Examen*, 322n1. "He aqui una razon entre mil que pudieran darse contra nobleza hereditaria, pues de ser un hombre grande quien formó una gerarquia, no se sigue que lo serán sus sucesores; asi lo natural es que la nobleza fuese adquirida personal- mente, es decir, por acciones laudables grandes en favor de su patria, no por pergaminos mas ó menos viejos, que servirán mucho cuando se trate de los origenes de las familias de sus anti- guos timbres, pero de nada debieran valer cuando los sucesores de un héroe son holgazanes é inhábiles."

76. Sánchez Villa, *Entre materia y espíritu*, 560.

77. Vázquez García, *La invención del racismo*, 211n10. While the Spanish case was unique, similar rhetoric circulated throughout Europe during the period; see Pick, *Faces of Degenera- tion*.

78. Rohr, "Philosephardism and Antisemitism in Turn-of-the-Century Spain," 376.

79. Martínez y Fernández, *Espejo del verdadero médico*, v: "Aunque rabino soy tolerante, y tanto, que habiendo traducido integro el segundo libro de esta obra de un autor católico, no quise molestarme en rehacerle respecto á lo que dice de la religion del médico."

80. Ibid., 10: "deseáramos que supiese el árabe para desenterrar antiguos monumentos de glorias patrias"; "francés es el comun de las naciones, es la lengua de los sábios contempora- neos, como Paris es la Atenas de los tiempos modernos."

81. Ibid., 12: "dedicarse exclusiva y concienzudamente al estudio del hombre en su estado físico, intelectual, y moral."

82. While at first glance it may seem strange that Martínez managed to combine positive eugenics with philosemitism, this was not an uncommon combination. See Rohr, "Philosephardism and Antisemitism in Turn-of-the-Century Spain."

83. Friedman, "Recovering Jewish Spain," 20.

84. Puigblanch [Natanael Jomtob], *La Inquisición sin máscara.*

85. The conservative vision of an "eternal Spain," compromised by religious pluralism but heroically revived via the Reconquest, has been remarkably durable. In June 2022, Giorgia Meloni, the leader of the Brothers of Italy, a party descended from the fascist Italian Social Movement, declared in a speech to the far-right Spanish party Vox, that, "Five hundred years ago, the capitulation of Granada put an end to the Reconquista, Andalucia turned Spanish, and Europe became Christian. Today the secularism of the left and radical Islam threaten our roots" (quoted in Yascha Mounk, "Italians Didn't Exactly Vote for Fascism").

86. Pulido Fernández, *Espanoles sin patria y la raza sefardi,* 50, quoted in Rohr, "Philosephardism and Antisemitism in Turn-of-the-Century Spain," 378. Michael Friedman discusses Pulido at length in chapter 4, "Reclaiming Sepharad: Spain's Jewish Past Between *Sefardismo* and *Hispanidad*" ("Recovering Jewish Spain").

87. Martínez y Fernández, *Espejo del verdadero médico,* vi: "Judio como soy, hablando de los autores españoles, les llamo nuestros, porque desciendo por linea recta de los Maimones de Lara de España; y aunque, como judio, errante y sin patria, llevo y tengo siempre á España por la mia."

88. Suárez de Ribera, *Medicina ilustrada chymica observada o theatros pharmacologicos, medico practicos, chymico-galenicos.*

89. Ibid., 17: "la Medicina . . . ha caído tanto, por algunos individuos, que la exercen, que son Judios; pues estos, como enemigos nuestros, toman este empleo, para tener mas ocasion de ofender à Christo, y à los Christianos."

90. Ibid., 20: "sin duda serian totalmente destruidos los Judios Medicos, si el Santo Tribunal de la Inquisition obligasse à qualquiera, que huviesse de exercer la Medicina, ò la Cirugia, &c. . . . presentassen los referidos instrumentos ante dicho Tribunal, y en este dados por buenos passassen al Real Proto-Medicato."

91. Martínez y Fernández, *Espejo del verdadero médico,* v: "salir a la defensa de mis hermanos los medicos rabinos contra Suárez Rivera, que le plugo pintarnos de este modo: 'Son los medicos judios llanos, aparentes, soberbios y aduladores.'"

92. Ibid., vi: "Aunque bien visto, no dejan hoy de tener esos mismos vicios los médicos cristianos."

93. Ibid., 93: "[L]a religion del médico es la *humanidad:* religion universal que, basada en el hombre, objeto de su estudio y de sus meditaciones, no puede menos de ser *tolerante* con todas, y por lo mismo, sea cualquiera la que profese el médico, llegará á, cumplir con su deber si sabe ser religioso, esto es, *humano,* caritativo en toda la estension de la palabra; *in omnibus charitas,* que dijo San Agustin."

94. Ibid., 107: "Esta fuera de confesion, escomulgado, el médico que no asiste a los apestados con peligro de su vida, aun cuando no esté asalariado, y aunque no perciba por sus visitas estipendio alguno, pues es el acto mas grande y sublime de su digno ministerio, y quien á él falta no debe condecorarsele con el nombre de médico."

95. Torrecilla, *España al revés,* 51.

5. Spain in the Time of Cholera

1. "Desengaños y esperanzas," *El Siglo Médico*, January 7, 1855, 1: "¡Año bajo muchos aspectos azaroso! ; año fecundo en risueñas ilusiones, pero tambien en amarguisimos desengaños!"

2. Ibid.: "como todo lo que en el interior puede conducir á la conservacion de la salud pública."

3. Ibid.: "Merecen en este sitio mencion especial los servicios eminentes de los compañeros que han tenido la gloriosa pero desgraciada suerte de luchar contra el destructor monstruo que abortaran las cenagosas orillas del Ganges."

4. Ibid.: "¡Cuanto heroismo por su parte, cuánta abnegacion, cuánto valor y cuánto desinteres! Pero ¡qué olvido, qué desprecio tan humillante por parte del Gobierno!

5. López Piñero, introduction to *La ciencia en la España del siglo XIX*, 16. See also Albarracín Teulón, "Las asociaciones médicas en España del siglo XIX," 135–38.

6. Valenzuela Calendario, "El espejismo del ejercicio libre," 273.

7. *El Siglo Médico* 1 (January 1, 1854): 6: "Cuando el arreglo de partidos está ya hace mucho tiempo durmiendo en el ministerio de la Gobernacion, ¿qué poder, qué influencia, qué fatalidad le detiene para que no salga á luz? No lo sabemos; pero estamos persuadidos que *si los sugetos citados quisiesen, ya estaria publicado,* ya estarian mis *representados* gozando de su benefica influencia; y esto es tan cierto, que no será la *impotencia* de la clase la que le tiene dormido y sin curso, sino la *apatia,* la *inaccion* de estas *lumbreras* de la ciencia."

8. Ibid.: "el ilustrado y laborioso médico D. Ildefonso Martínez." "Ardua empresa es la de penetrar las intenciones de un escritor; pero, si no fueren conocidos los deseos sanísimos y el leal proceder del autor de la epístola, acaso no faltase quien se sintiera inclinado a creer que llevaba en los párrafos transcritos el doble objeto de adquirir popularidad al paso que con un garbo y una donosura capaces de cautivar los corazonez mas empedernidos, procuraba *echar el muerto al vecino,* como suele decirse."

9. Ibid.: "Que sale bien la cosa. . . . Pues entonces nosotros lo hemos hecho: ¡ya se estaba ahogando el pobrecito arreglo de partidos, y tuvimos la caridad de sacarle de entre el fango y las arenas del mar!—Al contrario, que sale mal. . . . En ese caso es que *no han querido* los sugetos citados, las *lumbreras,* para que nos entendamos; es que han sido *impotentes* (¡uf!) *apáticos* ó *inactivos.*"

10. Ibid.: "es la verdad que varios médicos notables y de influencia han interpuesto y estan interponiendo cada dia sus buenos oficios para que se publique cuanto antes el proyecto que un alto cuerpo consultivo tiene presentado."

11. Ibid., 7: "Sin necesidad de *comités,* de agitacion intempestiva y arriesgada."

12. Rivadeneyra, *Arreglo de los partidos médicos.*

13. *El Crisol* 3: 10: "Hicísteis un arreglo de partidos que costó grandes trabajos, y que por ser resultado de un gobierno, sin la iniciativa de la clase, cayó anatemizado por los pueblos y derruido por las voces y gritería de una revolucion política."

14. *El Crisol* 2: 16: "Parece que los médicos españoles tratan de celebrar una junta magna con el objeto de designar á los individuos de la aristocracia médica que merezcan el *capelo de cardenal,* por sus predicaciones cerca del Gobierno para mejorar el estado de la clase."

15. See chapter 1, above.

16. Albarracín Teulón describes this episode in "Las asociaciones médicas en España del siglo XIX," 137–38.

17. *El Siglo Médico* 2 (January 8, 1854): 11, quoted by Albarracín Teulón, "Las asociaciones médicas en España del siglo XIX," 137: "El pensamiento de establecer en Madrid un *Colegio médico,* es un pensamiento elevado y digno que a todo trance debemos realizar. Con ese colegio, que pudieramos llamar central, se relacionarian facilmente los colegios médicos que á su sombra deberán aparecer en las capitales de las provincias, y comunicando con estos los profesores de los partidos resulla-ria una organizacion medica y completa. Demos principio por el centro. Brindemos por el pronto establecimiento de un *Colegio médico* en la capital de España."

18. Manuel Chust Calero and Juan Marchena Fernández take issue with characterizations of the Liberal Triennial as "parenthetical" in the introduction to *Los ecos de Riego en el mundo hispano (1820–1825)*.

19. See Rújula López and Chust Calero, eds., *El Trienio Liberal,* and Zozaya, "Moral Revenge of the Crowd." An even more ambitious attempt to reframe the francocentric conventional wisdom on the Revolutionary Era is Isabella, *Southern Europe in the Age of Revolutions.*

20. For further historiographic contextualization of the Revolution of 1854, see Pablo Sánchez León's introduction to Sánchez León and Labrador Méndez, *Las jornadas de julio (de 1854).* For general overviews of the revolutionary biennial, see Kiernan, *La revolucion de 1854 en España;* Bahamonde Magro and Martínez Martín, *Historia de España. Siglo XIX,* 303–36; and Esdaile, *Spain in the Liberal Age,* 97–103.

21. On the role of the "Hymn to Riego" in revolutionary political culture, see Moreno Luzón and Núñez Seixas, *Los colores de la patria.*

22. Un hijo del pueblo, 97: "De modo que Madrid en su totalidad era un campo de batalla; en todas partes corría sangre, en todas partes retumbaban las detonaciones de las descargas y el estampido de los cañonazos. Los hospitales de sangre, tanto de los paisanos como los de la tropa, recibían sin cesar heridos; aquí y allá era frequente ver un cadáver abandonado ya de la tropa ya de los paisanos."

23. Esdaile, *Spain in the Liberal Age,* 104–5.

24. Martínez y Fernández, "Carta de un sordo-mudo al General Espartero," 1.

25. Ibid., 1 (pagination mine): "Yo, Señor Escmo, soy sordo, y como tal, despreciaré necesariamente rumores que no he de oir, murmuraciones que no he de entender, criticas que el balde me harán, porque sordo á todo, siguiré mi camino con nobleza é independencia."

26. Ibid., 2: "mudo para la calumnia, mudo para la asechanza, mudo para la deshonra."

27. Ibid., 2–3: "no han penetrado en mi mente mas que las ideas puras, absolutas, y por tanto mi intuicion y mi estudio me han dado a conocer lo que valen las revoluciones, lo que prestan los revolucionarios."

28. Ibid., 3: "Si, Escmo Señor, estaís rodeado de asechanzas, acariciado por enemigos, adormecido por los laureles, y envanecido con la victoria, y sin embargo hay tanto que hacer."

29. Ibid.: "hay muchos que cuidar y nos hemos sentado tan presto; hay tanto que destruir y nos hemos fastidiado tan pronto; hay mucho que saber, y no hemos aprendido nada, ni aun en la desgracia; hay mascaras que arrancar, y dejamos que todos bailen cubiertos con la careta de libertad."

30. Ibid., 4: "Los proclamados liberales . . . quieren hoy profanar tambiien el arbol santo de la libertad, á cuyo sombra le han acogido."

31. Ibid.: "Ojo, alerta liberales, alerta Espartero, la marcha del año cuarenta y tres sea leccion severa, aprended siquiera una vez a no ser debiles ni generosos con vuestros enemigos!

. . . Ojala pudieramos tener un Wassington! pero á pesar del orgullo de muchos pretendidos grandes hombres, la España actual es el pais de Lilipud, no existen mas que enanos. Enanos en política, enanos en literatura, enanos revolucionarios."

32. Ibid., 5: "no es la epoca normal, la epoca es revolucionaria y revolucionaria progresiva, hoy mas liberal que ayer, mañana mas que hoy."

33. Ibid.: "he aprendido con la soledad, con el estudio, con la experiencia, que la quietud, que la tolerancia, que el osculo de paz dado a los traidores, no sirve sino para envanecerlos y en valen tomarlos, para que se burlen de nosotros, para que nos escarnezcan, para que nos compadezcan por tontos, porque no hay tonteria mayor que dar muestra á nuestros enemigos para tener despues el gusto de hacer los martires, esta es . . . una tonteria liberal."

34. Ibid., 6: "Es grande error, Escmo Sr., es grave culpa la de los titulados progresistas temer tanto un arbol que tan buenos y sazonados frutos da, y es un error gravisísimo, en hombres como Espartero temer la libertad, de la que no puede sino esperar bienes, y no temer al despotismo de quien seguramente solo puede esperar el cadalso."

35. Ibid., 8: "no y eternamente no, el inmortal Riego, el desgraciado Laci, el valiente Porlier os dicen de la tumba 'Aprende, aprende, librate pronto, no seas obstinado como nosotros, no fies en halagueñas promesas, pues cuando quieras recordar, será ya tarde, muy tarde, te vendras a reducir fuera de tiempo, y como el topo no sabras abrir los ojos sino para tu perdicion! . . .'

Zurbano clama desde la tumba 'Yo peleé por el trono y la constitucion ¿que hizo de mí ese trono, que ha hecho de mí el despotismo? . . . un martir.' Abrid, Escmo Sr., vuestros ojos a la razon, no temais la libertad, no la comprimais, dejad que todos enseñen, que todos doctrinen ¿que perderais con los ultra-liberales? Nada, absolutamente nada, antes bien ganarias lo que no puedes ganar marcando el paso."

36. Ibid.: "os han expatriado, os han secuestrado y reducido a la nulidad en Logroño, si siendo atentos, han sufrido los liberales todos los daños imaginables. harán mas de vosotros si teneis el valor bastante para llevar la revolucion á sus ultimas y mas logicas consecuencias?"

37. Ibid.: "si Riego dia 4 de julio hubiese con su prestigio dirijido al pueblo y ahorcado á un rey perjuro, hubiera sufrido mayor castigo que ser ahorcado? No ciertamente, y el murió ahorcado, por no haber tenido el valor de ahorcar, á quien en ley debió de hacerlo si hubiera sido revolucionario; no lo fué, y murió sin embargo ahorcado y arrastrado en un serón el que tres años antes había sido conducido en triunfo y tirado su carro por generales."

38. Ibid., 9: "el despotismo no mirará si has sido mas ó menos liberal, sino que has vivido un enemigo."

39. Ibid.: "esta es la que odian los tiranos y sus parciales."

40. Ibid., 9–10: "Si hubieras roto con el trono, con valor con energia revolucionaria, no hubieras sido desterrado, quisistes contemporizar, quisistes respetar, y la institucion venció al hombre debil, como hubiera sido vencido por el hombre fuerte ya se llamase Cromuel ó Napoleon."

41. Ibid., 10: "la situacion es la misma, la lucha es la eterna, el rey contra el pueblo."

42. Ibid., 11–12: "Escucha, General Espartero, escucha una vez siquiera la voz de la razon, no seas tan generoso, no fies tanto en sus fuerzas y las de tu partido, desconfia de muchos que te rodean, haz una guerra franca a la apostasia, libranos de tanta sangrijuela del estado, castiga los presupuestos ponte resueltemente de parte del contribuyente y no del empleado, da un gobierno justo y barato y merecerás nuestro para bien y el de la nacion entera. Pero si te

confias como en el año cuarenta y tres: si atiendes á los empleados y te falta valor para hacer reformas radicales, escucha tambien, tu porvenir: tu prestigio perderá de día en día, porque obras son amores y no buenas razones: dejarás de ser aclamado, porque si las reformas las dejas á tus nietos, no querran los que hoy viven tener tanta paciencia para esperar: serás responsable ante dios y los hombres, de no haber hecho nada, cuando podias hacerlo todo: serás tachado en la historia como un hombre subalterno de corto entendimiento y de menos valor, y todo tu prestigio y gloria y patriotismo ser á calificado como gloria vana."

43. Martínez y Fernández,. "Discurso pronunciado por D. Ildefonso Martínez en el aniversario de la muerte de D. Rafael del Riego," "Pueblo de Madrid, pueblo victorioso y heroico de los dias 18, 19 y 20 de julio": "Contemplad, ciudadanos, este catafalco colocado en el sitio del ignominioso patibulo, mirad ese retrato y esos trofeos, que no son mas que la apoteosis de un martir de la libertad, de una de las muchas victimas de la tirania de Fernando." On the role of martyred heroes in general, and Riego in particular, in the construction of a progressive political culture, see Zurita Aldeguer, "El progresismo," 320–46.

44. Martínez y Fernández, "Discurso pronunciado por D. Ildefonso Martínez en el aniversario de la muerte de D. Rafael del Riego": "Apercibid todos en este triste ejemplo, la veleidad de la fortuna, el rencor de los tiranos, la fuerza y la violencia ejercida contra los libres. Escuchad, patriotas, el pago que los reyes dan á sus leales servidores."

45. Ibid.: "ha[n] hecho mas daño que los mismos realistas."

46. Martínez y Fernández, El Crisol 3 (1855): 5: "En efecto, apareció el mes de enero de 1854 con un periódico nuevo, hijo natural y de legítimo matrimonio del anciano Boletin y de la jovenzuela Gaceta, y el niño se bautizó Siglo Médico. . . . creceria robusto y pelaria como camorrista con todo el mundo, si bien guardando las reglas de la decencia por ser órgano oficial de la burocracia médica."

47. "Exámen necesario," El Siglo Médico 27 (July 2, 1854): 215.

48. El Porvenir Médico 97 (August 5, 1854): 169: "Brevemente, y con el solo objeto de satisfacer una justa reclamacion de varios comprefesores, vamos á ocuparnos de otra nuevo atentado perpetrado por El Siglo Médico, contra la principal inmunidad de la clase. Doloroso nos es, hoy mas que nunca, tener que poner nuevamente en evidencia los desmanes del periódico polaco, los instintos ruines de esos hombres reaccionarios."

49. Ibid., 169–70: "Vivan tranquilos los profesores de Vigo y todos aquellos contra quienes el periódico polaco desató su enojo; ya pasaron aquellos tiempos para no volver; hoy no se recojen los periódicos ni se atropellan las personas por complacer a los bajos aduladores del poder; hoy están entronizadas la justicia y la moralidad que tanto asustan á ciertos hombres, por mas que para medrar aparenten rendirlas culto con refinada hipocresia; vivan tranquilos los que todo lo temieron de las tenebrosas maquinaciones del club médico, que hor no se sofoca el pensamiento; pero queden esculpidas en las mente de todos los profesores las palabras de el Siglo, para arrojarselas á la cara cuando cacaree, como acosturmbra su entusiasmo pro la profesion que rebaja, humila y degrada."

50. El Siglo Médico 30 (July 30, 1854): 233: "En los momentos mismos en que los combatientes, ciegos por el furor que los agita ó entusiasmados por la santidad de la causa que defienden, solo piensan en dañarse y destruirse mútuamente; allí donde las mas terribles pasiones apenas dejan lugar á la reflexion; allí donde reinan el ódio y la venganza con todo su terrifico aparato, se presenta un hombre sereno y tranquilo, lleno de caridad, de amor y de

ciencia, esponiéndose inerme á los estragos del plomo mortífero para arrebatarle sus víctimas, para llevar el consuelo á los vencidos y aplacar el rigor de los vencedores. Este hombre es el médico-cirujano."

51. Ibid.: "¡Ah! que la medicina es la segunda religion de la humanidad y los que la ejercen son sacerdotes consagrados á la práctica de la mas sublime virtud de la religion verdadera."

52. Ibid.: "¡Que los pueblos se penetren de esta importante verdad, y agradecida la sociedad sabrá compensar con su consideracion á los que tan alto rayan en el campo de la civilizacion y de la moral!"

53. On these efforts see Callahan, "Church and State, 1808–1874."

54. *El Siglo Médico* 30 (July 30, 1854): 255: "¿No vemos al gobierno dispensar especial proteccion al estado eclesiástico, ordenando las cosas de manera que el número de clérigos se ajuste á las necesidades, y procurando que no pueda faltarles la decorosa subsistencia que aquel estado reclama para llenar cumplidamente su alta mision?"

55. Ibid.: "¿No vemos intervenir debidamente al gobierno en la enseñanza primaria, determinando las cualidades que los maestros han de reunir, autorizandoles para la enseñanza, señalando sus asignaciones etc.?"

56. Ibid.: "Sin esta protection las clases médicas muy dificilmente serán a la sociedad todo lo utiles que pueden y deben ser." "los hombres ocupados incesantemente en la asistencia de los enfermos, sin defensa contra los miasmas pestilenciales, sin descanso, sin hora de placer."

57. *El Porvenir Médico* 95 (July 25, 1854): 161: "Creeriamos faltar á nuestros mas impres-cindibles deberes, si no nos ocuparamos, aunque de paso, de la gloriosa revolucion política que estamos atravesando, revolucion que ocupará un distinguido lugar en los fastos de la historia y que colocará nuestra patria á la altura de las naciones mas adelantadas en civilizacion y cultura, si la marcha ulterior de los acontecimientos no la desvia del magestuoso rumbo que ha emprendido. La revolucion actual no es de un partido; es un alzamiento nacional en que el honor y la dignidad de todos los españoles honrados se ha levantado contra la inmoralidad y la prevaricacion de los gobernantes; es el pensamiento oprimido que ha roto sus cadenas; es la libertad política que ha sepultado á la tirania; es el derecho triunfante contra la fuerza; es por fin, la restauracion del principio de la LEY y de la MORAL."

58. Ibid.: "Para lograr la regeneracion del cuerpo médico, como la del cuerpo físico, es necesario hacer un esmerado diagnóstico, investigar escrupulosamente todos los elementos patológicos de la dolencia, medir con exactitud su fuerza y malignidad, buscar en la terapéu-tica el oportuno remedio y aplicarle resueltamente, con criterio pero sin temor, con juicio pero con valentia."

59. Ibid., no. 96 (July 31, 1854): 161: "esta obra es la que deben proseguir hoy con incansable ardor; es preciso inculcar en el pueblo las ideas de libertad, es necesario esplicarle lo que no entiende, es indispensable demonstrarle lo erróneo de las preoccupaciones de que malevol-amente le han nutrido." This image of the evangelizing physician was nothing new; Michel Foucault describes how in the wake of the French Revolution there emerged a "myth of a nationalized medical profession, organized like the clergy, and invested, at the level of man's bodily health, with powers similar to those exercised by the clergy over men's souls" (*The Birth of the Clinic*, 31).

60. *El Porvenir Médico* no. 96 (July 31, 1854): 165: "De esta manera, no solamente prestarán las clases facultativas un bien incalculable al pais, sino que acrecerá la importancia social de

la medicina y llegarán sus professores á influir directa y poderosamente en la administracion del pais, unico medio de que la ciencia sea apreciada en todo su valor y de que las reformas que la profesion exija se soliciten dignamente desde los escaños del parlamento, y no desde las antesalas de las oficinas ministeriales."

61. Ibid., 165–66: "venimos oponiendo un dique moral á sus desmesuradas ambiciones y á sus tenebrosos planes; esa falange que acude a presurosa á cortar el paso á la juventud, valiéndose de reprobados manejos, no será estraño que defienda la reaccion para defender sus sueldos; mas si esto sucede seremos mas esplicitos y haremos conocer la verdad á la clase, sin mas que llamar cada hombre y cada cosa por su nombre."

62. Ibid., no. 108 (September 30, 1854): 213–14: "*¿En que pais vivimos?*—.... Hemos hablado con un gran número de profesores, y todos nos preguntan atónitos ¿es posible que esto diga un gobierno liberal, obra de la revolucion de julio, en cuya bandera teñida con la sangre del pueblo se leian las preciosas palabras *libertad, moralidad?*"

63. Ibid.: "nuestros compañeros que espontaneamente se hubieran sacrificado por salvar las vidas de los enfermos . . . sin amenanzas de castigos ridículos."

64. Ibid.: "Oblige el gobierno á todos los médicos que sean empleados suyos; castiguelos en buen hora el dia que abandonando sus puestos falten á su deber, supuesto que les proporciona una decorosa substistencia . . . pero déjenos á nostros que nada recibimos de él, respete siquiera nuestra libertad personal, ya que ninguna consideracion merecemos."

65. Ibid.: "No pretendemos atacar ni defender la marcha política de uno y otro gobierno, pues en ambos la encontramos mala y defectuosa."

66. Esdaile, *Spain in the Liberal Age,* 106.

67. Ibid.

68. On this counterrevolution, see Fontana i Làzaro, *La época del liberalismo,* 282–89.

69. *Gaceta Médica,* April 10, 1850, 163: "Dignos son por cierto de llamar la atención estos ejercicios, ahora que tan raros se van haciendo los de su especie, con grave perjuicio de la ciencia y de la profesión."

70. Ibid.: "conocidos todos, y notables, no solamente por su ilustración, pero también por la severidad de sus principios, la independencia é imparcialidad de su caracter."

71. *Boletin de Medicina, Cirugía, y Farmacia,* May 26, 1850, 167: "Solamente es de lamentar que no haya obtenido colocacion el Sr. D. Ildefonso Martínez que ocupaba el primer lugar para los baños de Buyeres de Nava; porque si dignos son los dos comprofesores agraciados, no lo es menos por cierto este joven ilustrado y erudito. Esperamos todavia que el Gobierno, justo apreciador de sus merecimientos, busque algun medio de utlizar tan buena disposicion."

72. *Gaceta Médica,* May 30, 1850, 208: "De resultas de esta eleccion ha quedado sin colocacion al aventajado joven D. Ildefonso Martínez, que ademas de estar propuesto en primer lugar para los baños de Buyeres habia hecho otras muchas oposiciones con igual aprovechamiento. El gobierno, que habrá tenido sus razones para preferir al Sr. Mestre, creemos no haya encontrado ninguna que haga desmerecer al Sr. Martínez del lugar que ha ganado en público certamen, y por lo tanto se halla en cierto modo obligado, para proceder lógica y equitativamente, á indemnizarle del perjuicio que sin culpa suya ha sufrido, concediéndole alguna otra vacante en el mismo ramo, sin necesidad de nuevos ejercicios de oposicion."

73. Ibid., March 30, 1851, 71.

74. Martínez y Fernández, *Espejo del verdadero médico,* 191: "Que las oposiciones tienen

defectos capitales en el orden con que hoy se efectúan, es cosa demostrada, esta fuera de toda duda; pero aun a pesar de sus inconvenientes, son preferibles a la eleccion por parte del gobierno."

75. Ibid., 194: "Otra objecion contra las oposiciones son los desafueros que suelen ejecutar los que gobiernan, nombrando al segundo ó tercero que va en terna, y dejando sin plaza al que va en primer lugar."

76. Ibid., 195: "esta reforma es la necesidad de que la prensa médica, la prensa científica, se ocupe en cada uno de sus números de dar el fallo acerca del mérito de los actos"; "la independencia de los periodistas, que si estuviese en uso tendrian mucha cuenta de no aventurar jucios temerarios, sino mas bien ser los fieles intérpretes de la opinion pública."

77. González Quiros, "El Dr. D. Ildefonso Martínez y Fernández," 79.

78. *El Siglo Médico* 76 (June 17, 1855): 185: "Dicho señor diputado, ardiente defensor de los intereses mercantiles, ha conseguido como por sorpresa de las Córtes españolas la anulacion de nuestro sistema cuarentanario completo."

79. Ibid., 187: "De todos modos la España queda abierta en adelante para el cólera morbo, y por lo tanto muchos millares de españoles pagarán con la vida las escasisimas ventajas que pueda reportar el comercio."

80. Ibid., no. 80 (July 15, 1855): 217: "¿Qué hacen pues las naciones de la culta Europa en presencia de un azote que las empobrece y despuebla? Apáticas, indiferentes, ocupadas en mortíferas guerras, dominadas por la política que es la mania del siglo, porque cada siglo tiene su peculiar mania, ávidas al propio tiempo de esa fácil y pronta riqueza que proporciona la libertad mercantil, al paso que olvidadizas de que el hombre es el primero y mas principal elemento de riqueza, como que es quien produce con su entendimiento y con sus brazos, apenas adoptan contra aquel alguna medida higiénica las mas veces de problemática eficacia."

81. On the contentious issues of contagion and quarantine, see Arrizabalaga and García-Reyes, "Contagion Controversies on Cholera and Yellow Fever in Mid Nineteenth-Century Spain."

82. *El Crisol* 16 (1855): 13–14: "Somos contagionistas, no por capricho, por mera induccion, sino por esperiencia práctica: hemos estado seis meses luchando con el cólera . . . y seguido en su marcha con interes y sin miedo, y aunque nuestra pequeñez cientifica sea de poco valer á los ojos de hombres eminentes . . . las cuarentenas marítimas, el acordonamiento fronterizo, corroboran las ideas contagionistas, y la última constelacion colérica francesa atrajo a nuestras banderas multitud de partidarios."

83. Hamlin, *Cholera: The Biography*, 5.

84. Moro, *Las epidemias de cólera en la Asturias del siglo XIX*, 44.

85. Libro de Acuerdos de 1855–1856, A-146, fols. 98v–99r, Archivo Municipal de Oviedo.

86. Ibid., fols. 99r–100r.

87. Ibid., fols. 101v–102r.

88. Martínez, *Cartilla popular higiénica y terapéutica del cólera morbo asiático*.

89. Libro de Acuerdos de 1855–1856, A-146, fols. 103r–v.

90. Ibid., fol. 108v.

91. Acta de la sesión del Ayuntamiento de 26/09/1855 (AMO. A-146 f. III r.–v). The death certificate erroneously reported his age as thirty-two.

92. See, for example, the biographical sketch that prefaces the catalog of his collected papers, BH Arch. IMF, 3.

93. *El Siglo Médico* 92 (October 7, 1855): 319–20: "Forzado por el gobernador de Oviedo á la asistencia de los coléricos . . . ha sido víctima de este procedimiento caprichoso y violento. . . . Si estuvieramos en un pais medianamente gobernado, no quedaria el gobernador de Oviedo sin sufrir una amarga represion por su proceder."

94. Ibid.: "La medicina patria ha perdido uno de sus mas entusiastas, apasionados, notable por su erudicion y estensos conocimientos. Nosotros tenemos la pena de haber perdido á una persona de quien siempre hemos hecho grande estima, por mas que se hubiese enfriado la amistad que algun dia nos profesó."

95. González Quiros, "El Dr. D. Ildefonso Martínez y Fernández," 79.

96. Libro de Acuerdos de 1855–1856, A-146, fols. iiir. –v, Archivo Municipal de Oviedo.

97. Ibid., fol. iiir: "El que suscribe tiene hoy el amargo sentimiento de anunciar á la Corporacion la sensible muerte del habil y pundonoroso facultativo D. Ildefonso Martínez, médico Director de los baños de Fuensanta, occurida á las tres de la madrugada de este dia, de resultas de un ataque fulminante de cólera. El Ayuntamiento tiene hoy un imperioso deber que cumplir, consagrando á la memoria del una logrado y distinguido profesor Martínez algun monumento que perpetue sus virtudes, su abnegacion y celo perseverante con que se ha dedicado al alivio y curacion de la desgraciada humanidad doliente."

Conclusion

1. Renders, "Exceptions That Prove the Rule," 69.

2. Grendi, "Micro-analisi e storia sociale," 506–20.

3. Loriga, "The Plurality of the Past," 34. Quoted in Meister, "The Biographical Turn and the Case for Historical Biography," 5.

4. Ibid., 39.

5. Meister, "The Biographical Turn and the Case for Historical Biography," 5.

6. Ibid., 6.

Bibliography

Primary Sources

ARCHIVAL SOURCES

Actas de la sesión del Ayuntamiento de Oviedo de 1855. Archivo Municipal de Oviedo.

Alcalá y Pavón, Bartolomé. "Fenómenos de la naturaleza." 1840. BH AP 4 leg. 1, doc. 20. UCM Biblioteca Histórica Marqués de Valdecilla.

Libro de Acuerdos de 1855–1856. Archivo Municipal de Oviedo.

Martínez y Fernández, Ildefonso. "El Archivo Personal de Ildefonso Martínez y Fernández." 1815–45. BH AP 4. Universidad Complutense de Madrid, Biblioteca Histórica Marqués de Valdecilla.

———. "Asilos de locos, e historia critica de la locura." June 1, 1846. BH AP 4, leg. 1, doc. 6. UCM Biblioteca Histórica Marqués de Valdecilla.

———. "Carta de un sordo-mudo al General Espartero." October 25, 1854. BH AP 4, leg. 3 doc. 1. UCM Biblioteca Histórica Marqués de Valdecilla.

———. "Compendio biográfico-bibliografico de la fisiologia." N.d. UCM Biblioteca Histórica Marqués de Valdecilla.

———. "Democracia, o El Porvenir." N.d. BH AP 4, leg. 3, doc. 5. UCM Biblioteca Histórica Marqués de Valdecilla.

———. "Discurso pronunciado por D. Ildefonso Martínez en el aniversario de la muerte de D. Rafael del Riego." November 1854. BH AP 4, leg. 3, doc. 2. UCM Biblioteca Histórica Marqués de Valdecilla.

———. "Disertacion leída al Ateneo Médico-Quirurjico Matritense." 1840. BH AP 4 leg. 1, doc. 7. UCM Biblioteca Histórica Marqués de Valdecilla.

———. "Del influjo de lo físico en lo moral y vice-versa." 1842. BH AP 4, leg. 1, doc. 6. UCM Biblioteca Histórica Marqués de Valdecilla.

———. "Los partidos." N.d. BH AP 4, leg. 3, doc. 6. UCM Biblioteca Histórica Marqués de Valdecilla.

———. "Proyecto de Una Emancipación Universal." May 5, 1847. BH AP 4 leg. 3. UCM Biblioteca Histórica Marqués de Valdecilla.

———. "Reglamento de la Sociedad Médico-Quirurgica de Emulación." 1839. BH AP 4 leg. 2, doc. 22. UCM Biblioteca Histórica Marqués de Valdecilla.

———. "Tratado de fisiología #1." N.d. BH AP 4, leg. 1, doc. 1. UCM Biblioteca Histórica Marqués de Valdecilla.

————. "Tratado de fisiología #2." N.d. BH AP 4, leg. 1, doc. 2. UCM Biblioteca Histórica Marqués de Valdecilla.

————. Universidades, 1225, exp. 8. Archivo Histórico Nacional, Madrid.

Romero Alpuente, Juan. "Sucesión á la corona de España." N.d. BH AP 4 leg. 3, doc. 7. UCM Biblioteca Histórica Marqués de Valdecilla.

PRINTED SOURCES

Acosta, Cristóbal. *Tratado en loor de las mujeres.* Venice: Imp. Iacomo Cornnetti, 1592.

Amich, Juan. *Acontecimientos políticos de la ciudad de Mataró en 1843 y sus consecuencias.* Mataró, 1855.

Barthez, Paul-Joseph. *Nouveaux éléments de la science de l'homme.* 2nd ed. Vol. 1. Paris, 1806.

Cabanis, P. J. G. [Pierre Jean Georges.] *On the Relations between the Physical and Moral Aspects of Man.* Ed. George Mora. Trans. Margaret Duggan Saidi. Baltimore: Johns Hopkins University Press, 1981.

Castro, Rodrigo de. *Medicus politicus.* Hamburg: Biblipolio Frobeniano, 1614.

Cerise, Laurent. *Exposé et examen critique du système phrénologique: considéré dans ses principes, dans sa méthode. . . .* Brussels: Société Typographique Belge, 1837.

Chinchilla Piqueras, Anastasio. *Anales históricos de la medicina en general y biográficos-bibliográficos de la española en particular.* Vol. 1. Valencia: Imprenta de López y Compañia, 1841.

————. *Historia de la medicina española.* Valencia, 1841.

Esquiros, Alphonse. *L'evangile du peuple.* Paris: Le Gallois, 1840.

————. *Histoire des martyrs de la liberté.* Paris: J. Bry aîné, 1851.

Fabra Soldevila, Francisco. *Filosofía de la legislación natural fundada en la antropología o en el conocimiento de la naturaleza del hombre y de sus relaciones con los demás seres.* Madrid: Imprenta del Colegio de Sordo-mudos, 1838.

Freyre de Castrillón, Manuel. *Contra el contrato social. Discurso segundo.* Santiago de Compostela: D. Juan Francisco Montero, 1810.

Gallardo, Bartolomé José. "Sensaciones." In *Diccionario de medicina y cirugía,* ed. Antonio Ballano, 64–77. Madrid: Imprenta Real, 1807.

————. "Sentidos." In *Diccionario de medicina y cirugía,* ed. Antonio Ballano, 93–100. Madrid: Imprenta Real, 1807.

Gallardo y Blanco, Bartolomé José. *Don Bartolomé José Gallardo, 1776–1852.* Ed. Antonio R. Rodríguez Moñino. Madrid: Sancha, 1955.

García Caballero, Félix. *De la libertad moral en sus relaciones con los delitos.* Madrid: Imprenta y libreria de D. Pedro Sanz y Sanz, 1854.

Hernández Morejón, Antonio. *Historia bibliográfica de la medicina española.* Biblioteca escojida de medicina y cirujía. Madrid: Impr. de la viuda de Jordan e hijos, 1842.

Hervás y Panduro, Lorenzo. *Carta Del Abate Don Lorenzo Hervás al Excelentísimo Señor Don Antonio Ponce de León. . . .* Madrid: Imprenta de la Administración del Real Arbitrio de Beneficencia, 1805.

Un hijo del pueblo. In *Las jornadas de julio (de 1854): (una crónica anónima de "otro" 15M en el pasado ciudadano español)*, ed. Pablo Sánchez León and Germán Labrador Méndez. Madrid: Postmetropolis Editorial, 2018.

Huarte de San Juan, Juan. *Examen de ingenios para las ciencias... Aumentado con las variantes de las más selectas ediciones y de su correspondiente juicio crítico.* Ed. Ildefonso Martínez y Fernández, Madrid, Imp. Primitivo Fuentes, 1845.

———. *Examen de ingenios para las ciencias, en el cual el lector hallará la manera de su ingenio para escoger la ciencia en que mas ha de aprovechar....* Ed. Ildefonso Martínez y Fernández. Madrid: Imprenta de D. Ramon Campuzano, 1846.

———. *Examen de ingenios para las ciencias.* Ed. Guillermo Serés. Madrid: Cátedra, 1989.

Janer, Félix. Gaceta Médica de Madrid. November 29, 1834, 26.

———. Gaceta Médica de Madrid. July 25, 1835, 8.

Jorge Enríquez, Enrique. *Retrato del perfecto médico.* Salamanca: Juan Andrés Renaut, 1595.

Llorente, Juan Antonio, and Gabriel H. Lovett. *A Critical History of the Inquisition of Spain: From the Period of Its Establishment by Ferdinand V to the Reign of Ferdinand VII....* Williamstown, MA: J. Lilburne Co., 1967.

López Mateos, Ramón. *Pensamientos sobre la razón de las leyes derivada de las ciencias físicas ó sea sobre la filosofía de la legislación.* Gómez Fuentenebro y Compañía, 1810.

Martínez y Fernández, Ildefonso [Dr. Barlo-Vento]. *La apología de los ciegos, ó la homeopato mania.* Madrid: Imprenta de Don José Trujillo, Hijo, 1851.

———. *Cartilla popular higiénica y terapéutica del cólera morbo asiático.* Oviedo: Comisión Facultativa de la Junta Provincial de Sanidad, 1855.

———[Rabbi Isaac Maimon Firdusi]. *Espejo del verdadero médico.* Madrid: Establecimiento Tipográfico de Don Andrés Peña, 1855.

———, "Las Historias de La Medicina de Chinchilla y Morejón." *Anales del Instituto Médico de Emulación. Periódico de Medicina, Cirugía, Farmacia y sus Ciencias Auxiliares* 48 (October 3, 1844): 380. www.filosofia.org/hem/184/8441003a.htm.

——— [El Doctor Palomeque]. *Médicos perseguidos por la Inquisición española.* Biblioteca del Crisol. Madrid: Establecimiento Tipográfico de D. Andrés Peña, 1855.

Masson de Morvilliers, Nicolas. "Espagne." In *Encyclopédie méthodique ou par ordre de matiéres,* series "Géographie modern." Vol. 1, 554–68.

Mata y Fontanet, Pedro. *Tratado de la razon humana con aplicacion á la prática del foro. Lecciones dadas en el Ateneo científico y literario de Madrid.* Madrid: C. Bailly-Bailliere, 1858.

———. *Filosofía española. Tratado de la razon humana con aplicacion á la prática del foro. Lecciones dadas en el Ateneo científico y literario de Madrid.* C. Bailly-Bailliere, 1858.

Merola, Jerónimo. *Republica original sacada del cuerpo humano.* Barcelona: Casa de Pedro Malo, 1587.

Monlau y Roca, Pedro Felipe. *Elementos de higiene pública.* Barcelona: Imprenta de D. Pablo Riera, 1847.

Mosácula, Juan. *Elementos de fisiología especial ó humana.* Vol. 2. Madrid, 1830.

Negrete, Cosme Gil. *Conclusiones medico politicae Philippo IIII hispaniarum regi catolico,* Madrid, 1654.

Pereira, Gómez. *Antoniana Margarita, Opus nempe physicis, medicis, ac theologis non minus utile, quam necessarium, per Gometium Pereiram, medicum Methinae Duelli, quae Hispanorum lingua Medina de el Campo appellatur, nunc primum in lucem aeditum.* Medina del Campo, 1554.

Programas para las asignaturas de segunda ensenanza mandadas observar por S. M. en todos los institutos, seminarios y colegios del reino por Real Orden de 20 de setiembre de 1850. Madrid, Imprenta Nacional, 1850.

Puigblanch, Antonio [Natanael Jomtob]. *La Inquisición sin máscara.* Cádiz, 1811.

Pulido Fernández, Ángel. *Espanoles sin patria y la raza sefardi.* Madrid, 1905.

Rivadeneyra, Manuel. *Arreglo de los partidos médicos.* Madrid: Imprenta y Estereotipía de M. Rivadeneyra, 1854.

Sabuco de Nantes Barrera, Oliva. *La nueva filosofía de la naturaleza del hombre, no conocida, ni alcanzada de los grandes filosofos antiguos, la qual mejora la vida, y salud humana.* Ed. Ildefonso Martínez y Fernández. Madrid: Colegio de Sordo-Mudos y Ciegos, 1847.

————, and Miguel Sabuco. *New Philosophy of Human Nature: Neither Known to nor Attained by the Great Ancient Philosophers. . . .* Ed. Mary Ellen Waithe, Mary Colomer Vintró, and C. Ángel Zorita. Urbana: University of Illinois Press, 2007.

Sabuco, Miguel, and Oliva Sabuco de Nantes y Barrera. *The True Medicine.* Ed. and trans. Gianna Pomata. Toronto: Iter, 2010.

Salvá, Jaime. "Observaciones sobre la obra titulada *Examen de ingenios* por Juan Huarte, escritor a fines del siglo XVI." *Revista de Madrid*, 3rd series, vol. 1 (1841): 266–76.

Suárez de Ribera, Francisco. *Medicina ilustrada chymica observada o theatros pharmacologicos, medico practicos, chymico-galenicos.* Madrid, 1725.

Varela de Montes, José, Ezequiel Martín de Pedro, Antonio Hernández Morejón, Antonio Fernández Carril, Eusebio Aguado, and Real Colegio de Cirugía de San Carlos (Madrid). *Ensayo de antropología ó sea historia fisiologica del hombre en sus relaciones con las ciencias sociales y especialmente con la patologia y la higiene.* Madrid: Imp. y fundición de Eusebio Aguado, 1844.

Villanueva, Joaquín Lorenzo. *Catecismo del Estado según los principios de la religión.* Madrid: Imprenta Real, 1793.

Volney, Constantin-François. *The Ruins: Or, Meditation on the Revolutions of Empires: And the Law of Nature.* New York: Peter Eckler Publishing Co., 1890.

PERIODICALS AND NEWSPAPERS

Anales del Instituto Médico de Emulación. Periódico de Medicina, Cirugía, Farmacia y sus Ciencias Auxiliares.

Boletín de Medicina, Cirugía, y Farmacia.

Boletín del Instituto Médico Valenciano.

Círculo Científico y Literario.

El Crisol. Floresta Crítica Médica.

Gaceta Médica de Madrid.

El Porvenir Médico.

Semanario Patriótico.

El Siglo Médico.

La Verdad. Periódico de Medicina y Ciencias Auxiliares.

Secondary Sources

Ackerknecht, Erwin H. *A Short History of Psychiatry.* Trans. Sula Wolff. New York: Hafner Publishing Co., 1968.

———. *Rudolf Virchow, Doctor, Statesman, Anthropologist.* Madison: University of Wisconsin Press, 1953.

Aguirre Marco, Carla Pilar. "Hernández Morejón, Anastasio Chinchilla y la historia de la medicina española." In *Hernández Morejón, Anastasio Chinchilla y la historia de la medicina española,* 121–98. Valencia: Universitat de València, 2008.

Albarracín Teulón, Agustín. "Las asociaciones médicas en España del siglo XIX." *Cuadernos de historia de la medicina Española* 10 (1971): 119–86.

———. "La profesión médica ante la sociedad española del siglo XIX." *Asclepio* 25 (1973): 303–16.

———. "La titulación médica en España durante el siglo XIX." *Cuadernos de Historia de la Medicina Espanola* 12 (1973): 15–79.

Alcalá, Ángel, ed. *The Spanish Inquisition and the Inquisitorial Mind.* Highland Lakes, NJ: Atlantic Research Publications, 1987.

Almagor, Laura, Haakon A. Ikonomou, and Gunvor Simonsen. *Global Biographies: Lived History as Method.* Manchester, UK: Manchester University Press, 2022.

Álvarez Junco, José. *Mater Dolorosa: la idea de España en el siglo XIX.* 14th ed. Madrid: Taurus, 2016.

———, and Adrian Shubert, eds. *Nueva historia de la España contemporánea (1808–2018).* Barcelona: Galaxia Gutenberg, 2018.

———, and Adrian Shubert, eds. *Spanish History since 1808.* London: Arnold, 2000.

Anderson, Benedict. *Imagined Communities: Reflections on the Origin and Spread of Nationalism.* London: Verso, 1983.

Anderson, Warwick, and Hans Pols. "Scientific Patriotism: Medical Science and National Self-Fashioning in Southeast Asia." *Comparative Studies in Society and History* 54, no. 1 (2012): 93–113.

Aresti Esteban, Nerea. "El ángel del hogar y sus demonios: ciencia, religión y genero en la España del siglo XIX." *Historia Contemporánea* 21 (2000): 363–94.

———. *Médicos, donjuanes y mujeres modernas: los ideales de feminidad y masculinidad en el primer tercio del siglo XX.* Bilbao: Universidad del País Vasco, 2001.

Arquiola, Elvira. "La incorporación a España de una visión utópica de la medicina." In *Ciencia en expansión: estudios sobre la difusión de las ideas científicas y médicas en España (siglos XVIII–XX),* ed. Elvira Arquiola and José Martínez Pérez, 105–19. Madrid: Universidad Complutense, 1995.

———, and Luis Montiel. *La corona de las ciencias naturales: la medicina en el tránsito del siglo XVIII al XIX.* Madrid: Consejo Superior de Investigaciones Científicas, 1993.

Arrizabalaga Valbuena, Jon. "The Ideal Medical Practitioner in Counter-Reformation Castile: The Perception of the Converso Physician Henrique Jorge Henriques (c. 1555–1622)." In *Medicine and Medical Ethics in Medieval and Early Modern Spain: An*

Intercultural Approach, ed. Samuel S. Kottek and Luis García Ballester, 61–91. Jerusalem: Magnes Press, 1996.

————. "Huarte de San Juan y la censura inquisitorial en la España de Felipe II." In *Pasados y presente: estudios para el profesor Ricardo García Cárcel,* edited by Rosa María Alabrús Iglesias et al., 583–94. Barcelona: Universitat Autónoma de Barcelona, Departament d'Història Moderna i Contemporània, 2020.

————, and Juan Carlos García-Reyes. "Contagion Controversies on Cholera and Yellow Fever in Mid Nineteenth-Century Spain: The Case of Nicasio Landa." In *Mediterranean Quarantines, 1750–1914: Space, Identity and Power,* ed. John Chircop and Francisco Javier Martinez, 170–95. Manchester, UK: Manchester University Press, 2018.

————, and Maria Laura Giordano. "Cristianismo Paulino en Huarte de San Juan: meritocracía y linaje en el Examen de ingenios para las ciencias (Baeza 1575, 1594)." *Hispania Sacra* 72, no. 146 (2020): 363–75.

Arroyo, Silvia. "Giving Birth to Science: Oliva Sabuco and Her Intrusions into the Male Episteme." In *Confined Women: The Walls of Female Space in Early Modern Spain,* ed. Brian M. Phillips and Emily Colbert Cairns, 90–109. Minneapolis: University of Minnesota Twin Cities, 2020. cla.umn.edu/hispanic-issues/online/confined-women-walls-female-space-early-modern-spain.

Artola, Miguel. *La burguesía revolucionaria (1808–1874).* Madrid: Alianza Editorial, 2006.

Bahamonde Magro, Ángel, and Jesús Antonio Martínez Martín. *Historia de España. Siglo XIX.* 3rd ed. Madrid: Cátedra, 2001.

Balltondre Pla, Mónica. "El conocimiento de sí y el gobierno de las pasiones en la obra de Sabuco." *Revista de Historia de la Psicología* 27, no. 2–3 (2006): 107–14.

Barnosell, Genís. "God and Freedom: Radical Liberalism, Republicanism, and Religion in Spain, 1808–1847." *International Review of Social History* 57, no. 1 (April 2012): 37–59.

Barona Vilar, Josep Lluis. *Sobre medicina y filosofía natural en el Renacimiento.* Valencia: Seminari d'Estudis sobre la Ciencia, 1993.

Benavente Barreda, José María. "Sensualismo." In *Encyclopedia de La Cultura Española* 5: 265–66. Madrid: Editora Nacional, 1968.

Bidwell-Steiner, Marlen. "Metabolisms of the Soul. The Physiology of Bernardino Telesio in Oliva Sabuco's Nueva Filosofía de La Naturaleza Del Hombre (1587)." In *Blood, Sweat and Tears: The Changing Concepts of Physiology from Antiquity into Early Modern Europe,* ed. Manfred Horstmanshoff et al., 661–83. Leiden: Brill, 2012.

Bolufer i Peruga, Mónica. "Cos femení, cos social. Apunts d'historiografia sobre els sabers médics i la construcció cultural d'identitats sexuades (segles XVI–XIX)." *Afers* 33–34 (1999): 531–50.

Boyd, Carolyn P. "The Military in Politics." In *Spanish History since 1808,* ed. Alvarez Junco and Shubert, 64–79.

Brooke, Elisabeth. *Women Healers Through History.* Aeon Books, 2020.

Bujosa Homar, Francesc. *Filosofía e historiografía médica en España: los supuestos epistemológicos de los historiadores clásicos de la medicina española.* Madrid: Consejo Superior de Investigaciones Científicas, 1989.

Burdiel, Isabel. "Historia política y biografía: más allá de las fronteras." In *Los retos de la biografía: la reflexion sobre la biografía se ha enriquecido en los últimos años...*, 47–83. *Ayer: Revista de Historia Contemporánea* 93, no. 1 (2014).

———. *Isabel II: una biografía (1830–1904)*. 6th ed. Madrid: Penguin Random House Group, 2018.

———. "The Liberal Revolution, 1808–1843." In *Spanish History since 1808*, ed. Alvarez Junco and Shubert, 17–32.

———. "*Los retos de la biografía: la reflexion sobre la biografía se ha enriquecido en los últimos años...*" *Ayer: Revista de Historia Contemporánea* 93, no. 1 (2014).

Bynum, W. F., Stephen Lock, and Roy Porter, eds. *Medical Journals and Medical Knowledge: Historical Essays*. New York: Routledge, 1992.

Caballé, Anna. "La biografía en España: primeras propuestas para la construcción de un canon." In *La historia biográfica en Europa: nuevas perspectivas*, ed. Isabel Burdiel, R. F. Foster, and Anaclet Pons, 89–117. Zaragoza: Institución Fernando el Católico, 2015.

Cabré, Monserrat, and Teresa Ortiz-Gómez, eds. "Mujeres y salud: prácticas y saberes / Women and Health: Practices and Knowledges." *Dynamis* 19 (1999).

Cabrera, Miguel Ángel. "El sujeto de la política: naturaleza humana, soberanía y ciudadanía." In Cabrera and Pro Ruiz, eds., *La creación de las culturas políticas*, 37–67.

———, and Juan Pro Ruiz, eds. *La creación de las culturas políticas modernas, 1808–1833*. Vol. 1: *Historia de las culturas políticas en España y América Latina*. Madrid: Marcial Pons Historia, 2014.

Caine, Barbara. *Biography and History*. 2nd ed. Basingstoke, Hampshire: Palgrave Macmillan, 2019.

Callahan, William J. "Church and State, 1808–1874." In *Nueva historia de la España contemporánea (1808–2018)*, ed. Alvarez Junco and Shubert, 48–63.

Campos Marín, Ricardo. *Monlau, Rubio, Giné: curar y gobernar: medicina y liberalismo en la España del siglo XIX*. Madrid: Nivola, 2003.

Carr, Raymond. *Spain, 1808–1975*. 2nd ed. Oxford, UK: Clarendon Press, 1982.

Castells, Irene. *La utopía insurreccional del liberalismo: Torrijos y las conspiraciones liberales de la década ominosa*. Barcelona: Editorial Crítica, 1989.

Castro Alfin, Demetrio. "Los ideólogos en España: La recepción de Destutt de Tracy y de Volny." *Estudios de Historia Social* 36–37 (1986): 337–43.

———. "The left: from liberalism to democracy." In *Spanish History since 1808*, ed. Alvarez Junco and Shubert, 79–90.

Cepedello Boiso, José. "La influencia de Condillac y los ideólogos en la teoría del derecho española decimonónica." In *La cultura del otro: Español en Francia, francés en España*, ed. Manuel Bruña Cuevas et al., 148–56. Sevilla: Universidad de Sevilla, 2006.

Checa Beltran, José. *Demonio y modelo. Dos visiones del legado español en la Francia ilustrada*. Madrid: Casa de Velázquez, 2014.

Chust Calero, Manuel, and Juan Marchena Fernández. *Los ecos de Riego en el mundo hispano (1820–1825)*. Madrid: Centro de Estudios Políticos y Constitucionales, 2022.

Cobb, Matthew. "A Brief History of Wires in the Brain." *Frontiers in Ecology and Evolution* 9 (2021). www.frontiersin.org/article/10.3389/fevo.2021.760269.

————. *The Idea of the Brain: The Past and Future of Neuroscience.* New York: Basic Books, 2020.

Cohen, William B. *The French Encounter with Africans: White Response to Blacks, 1530–1880.* Bloomington: Indiana University Press, 1980.

Coleman, William. *Biology in the Nineteenth Century: Problems of Form, Function, and Transformation.* Rpt. New York: Cambridge University Press, 1977.

Cruz, Jesús. "The Moderate ascendancy, 1843–1868." In *Spanish History since 1808,* ed. Alvarez Junco and Shubert, 33–47.

De Ceglia, Paolo Francesco. "Matter Is Not Enough: Georg Ernst Stahl, Friedrich Hoffman, and the Issue of Animism." *Journal of the International Society for the History of Philosophy of Science* 11, no. 2 (2021): 502–27.

Duffin, Jacalyn. "Vitalism and Organicism in the Philosophy of R.-T.-H. Laennec." *Bulletin of the History of Medicine* 62, no. 4 (Winter 1988): 525–45.

Dufour, Gérard. "Juan Antonio Llorente: de corifeo del afrancesamiento a mártir del liberalismo." *Ayer: Revista de Historia Contemporánea* 95, no. 3 (2014): 23–49.

Eastman, Scott. *Preaching Spanish Nationalism across the Hispanic Atlantic, 1759–1823.* Baton Rouge: Louisiana State University Press, 2012.

Eling, Paul, and Stanley Finger. *Franz Joseph Gall: Naturalist of the Mind, Visionary of the Brain.* Oxford, UK: Oxford University Press, 2019.

Elmer, Peter. *The Miraculous Conformist: Valentine Greatrakes, the Body Politic, and the Politics of Healing in Restoration Britain.* Oxford, UK: Oxford University Press, 2013.

Esdaile, Charles J. *Spain in the Liberal Age: From Constitution to Civil War, 1808–1939.* Oxford, UK: Blackwell Publishers, 2000.

Federspil, Giovanni, and Nicola Sicolo. "The Nature of Life in the History of Medical and Philosophic Thinking." *American Journal of Nephrology* 14, no. 4–6 (1994): 337–43.

Fernández-Medina, Nicolás. *Life Embodied: The Promise of Vital Force in Spanish Modernity.* Montreal: McGill-Queen's University Press, 2018.

Fernández Sarasola, Ignacio. *Los partidos políticos en el pensamiento español: De la Ilustración a nuestros días.* Madrid: Marcial Pons Historia, 2009.

Fernández Sebastián, Javier. "Periodismo." In *Diccionario político y social del siglo XIX español,* ed. Juan Francisco Fuentes and Javier Fernández Sebastián, 523–31. Madrid: Alianza Editorial, 2002.

Fontana i Làzaro, Josep. *La época del liberalismo.* Barcelona: Crítica, 2015.

Foucault, Michel. *The Birth of the Clinic: An Archaeology of Medical Perception.* New York: Vintage Books, 1994.

————. *The History of Sexuality.* 1st American ed. Vol. 1. New York: Pantheon Books, 1978.

————. *The Order of Things: An Archaeology of the Human Sciences.* New York: Vintage Books, 1973.

Friedman, Michael Rose. "Recovering Jewish Spain: Politics, Historiography and Institutionalization of the Jewish Past in Spain (1845–1935)." PhD diss., Columbia University, 2012.

Fuentes, Juan Francisco, and Javier Fernández Sebastián. "Liberalismo," in *Diccionario político y social del siglo XIX español,* ed. Juan Francisco Fuentes and Javier Fernández Sebastián. Madrid: Alianza Editorial, 2002.

García García, Emilio. "Huarte de San Juan, un adelantado a la teoría modular de la mente." *Revista de Historia de la Psicología* 24, no. 1 (2003): 9–25.

García Gómez, Mercedes Caridad. *La concepción de la naturaleza humana en la obra de Miguel Sabuco.* Albacete: Instituto de Estudios Alcacetenses, 1992.

García Guerra, Delfín, and Víctor Álvarez Antuña. *Lepra asturiensis: La contribución asturiana en la historia de la pelagra (siglos XVIII y XIX).* Oviedo: Universidad de Oviedo, 1993.

Giglioni, Guido. "Between Galen and St Paul: How Juan Huarte de San Juan Responded to Inquisitorial Censorship." *Early Science and Medicine* 23, no. 1–2 (2018): 114–34.

Gil Novales, Alberto. *El trienio liberal.* 1st ed. Madrid: Siglo XXI, 1980.

Ginger, Andrew, and Geraldine Lawless, eds. *Spain in the Nineteenth Century: New Essays on Experiences of Culture and Society.* Manchester, UK: Manchester University Press, 2018.

Ginsburg, Simona, and Eva Jablonka. *The Evolution of the Sensitive Soul: Learning and the Origins of Consciousness.* Cambridge, MA: MIT Press, 2019.

Goldstein, Jan. *Console and Classify: The French Psychiatric Profession in the Nineteenth Century.* Cambridge, UK: Cambridge University Press, 1987.

———. *Post-Revolutionary Self: Politics and Psyche in France, 1750–1850.* Cambridge, MA: Harvard University Press, 2005.

González, Román Miguel. *La pasión revolucionaria: Culturas políticas republicanas y movilización popular en la España del siglo XIX.* Madrid: Centro de Estudios Políticos y Sociales, 2007.

González Quiros Isla, Pedro. "El Dr. D. Ildefonso Martínez y Fernández. Una víctima del cumplimiento del deber. Un médico ilustre asiste a una epidemia de cólera." *Medicina Asturiana* 4 (April 1967): 75–99.

Gracia Guillén, Diego Miguel. "Ideología y ciencia clínica en la España de la primera mitad del siglo XIX." *Estudios de historia social* 12–13 (1980): 229–43.

———. "Judaism, Medicine, and the Inquisitorial Mind in Sixteenth-Century Spain." In *The Spanish Inquisition and the Inquisitorial Mind,* ed. Ángel Alcalá, trans. Esther da Costa-Frankel, 375–400. Highland Lakes, NJ: Atlantic Research Publications, 1987.

Granjel, Luis S. *Historia política de la medicina española.* Salamanca: Instituto de Historia de la Medicina Española, Universidad de Salamanca, 1985.

Grendi, Edoardo. "Micro-analisi e storia sociale." *Quaderni storici* 12, no. 35 (May–August 1977): 506–20.

Guerra, Francisco. "El exilio de médicos durante el siglo XIX." *Asclepio* 21 (1969): 223–48.

Gútiez, Carrión. "Ildefonso Martínez, amigo y bibliotecario de Gallardo." In *Homenaje a don Agustín Millares Carlo,* 557–65. Las Palmas de Gran Canaria: Caja Insular de Ahorros de Gran Canaria, 1975.

Guy, Alain. "Miguel Sabuco, psicólogo de las pasiones y precursor de la medicina psico-somática." *Al-Basit* 13, no. 22 (December 1987): 112–23.

Hagner, Michael. "Scientific Medicine." In *From Natural Philosophy to the Sciences: Writing the History of Nineteenth-Century Science,* ed. David Cahan, 49–87. Chicago: University of Chicago Press, 2003.

Haidt, Rebecca. "Emotional Contagion in a Time of Cholera: Sympathy, Humanity, and Hygiene in Mid-Nineteenth-Century Spain." In *Engaging the Emotions in Spanish Culture and History,* ed. Luisa Elena Delgado, Pura Fernández, and Jo Labanyi, 77–94. Nashville: Vanderbilt University Press, 2016.

Hajdu, Steven I. "Rudolph Virchow, Pathologist, Armed Revolutionist, Politician, and Anthropologist." *Annals of Clinical & Laboratory Science* 35, no. 2 (April 1, 2005): 203–5.

Haliczer, Stephen. "Inquisition Myth and Inquisition History: The Abolition of the Holy Office and the Development of Spanish Political Ideology." In *The Spanish Inquisition and the Inquisitorial Mind,* ed. Alcalá, 523–46.

Hall, Thomas S. *Ideas of Life and Matter: Studies in the History of General Physiology, 600 B.C.–1900 A.D.* Vol. 2. Chicago: University of Chicago Press, 1969.

Hamlin, Christopher. *Cholera: The Biography.* New York: Oxford University Press, 2009.

Harrington, Anne. *Medicine, Mind, and the Double Brain: A Study in Nineteenth-Century Thought.* Princeton, NJ: Princeton University Press, 1989.

Henares, D. *El bachiller Sabuco en la filosofía del Renacimiento español.* Albacete: Gráficas Panadero, 1976.

Herr, Richard. *The Eighteenth-Century Revolution in Spain.* Princeton, NJ: Princeton University Press, 1958.

Iriarte, Mauricio. *El doctor Huarte de San Juan y su Examen de ingenios. Contribución a la historia de la psicología diferencial.* Madrid: Jerarquía, 1939.

Isabella, Maurizio. *Southern Europe in the Age of Revolutions.* Princeton, NJ: Princeton University Press, 2023.

Jacobson, Steven, and Javier Moreno Luzón. "The Political System of the Restoration, 1875–1914: Political and Social Elites." In *Spanish History since 1808,* ed. Alvarez Junco and Shubert, 93–109.

Jacyna, L. S. "Medical Science and Moral Science: The Cultural Relations of Physiology in Restoration France." *History of Science* 25, no. 2 (1987): 111–46.

Kagan, Richard L. "Prescott's Paradigm: American Historical Scholarship and the Decline of Spain." *American Historical Review* 101, no. 2 (1996): 423–46.

———. *The Spanish Craze: America's Fascination with the Hispanic World, 1779–1939.* Lincoln: University of Nebraska Press, 2019.

———, ed. *Spain in America: The Origins of Hispanism in the United States.* Urbana: University of Illinois Press, 2002.

Kamen, Henry. *The Disinherited: Exile and the Making of Spanish Culture, 1492–1975.* New York: HarperCollins, 2007.

Keitt, Andrew. *Inventing the Sacred: Imposture, Inquisition, and the Boundaries of the Supernatural in Golden Age Spain.* Leiden: Brill, 2005.

———. "Medical Martyrs: Nineteenth-Century Representations of Early Modern Inquisitorial Persecution of Spanish Physicians." *Early Science and Medicine* 23, no. 1–2 (2018): 135–58.

———. "The Miraculous Body of Evidence: Visionary Experience, Medical Discourse, and the Inquisition in Seventeenth-Century Spain." *Sixteenth Century Journal* 36, no. 1 (2005): 77–96.

Kiernan, V. G. *La revolucion de 1854 en España.* Madrid: Aguilar, 1970.

Kimmel, Seth. "Tropes of Expertise and Converso Unbelief: Huarte de San Juan's History of Medicine." In *After Conversion,* ed. Mercedes García-Arenal, 336–57. Leiden; Boston: Brill, 2016.

Laín Entralgo, Pedro. *La edad de plata de la cultura española (1898–1936).* Madrid: Espasa Calpe, 1993.

Lakoff, George, and Mark Johnson, *Metaphors We Live By. Chicago: University of Chicago Press, 1981.*

Laqueur, Walter. "The Origins of Guerrilla Doctrine." *Journal of Contemporary History* 10, no. 3 (1975): 341–82.

Latour, Bruno. *We Have Never Been Modern.* Cambridge, MA: Harvard University Press, 1993.

Llorens, Vicente, and Andrés Amorós. *Liberales y románticos: Una emigración española en Inglaterra (1823–1834).* Valencia: Biblioteca valenciana, 2006.

López Piñero, José María. "Las ciencias médicas en la España del siglo XIX." In *La ciencia en la España del siglo XIX,* ed. José María López Piñero, 193–240. Madrid: Marcial Pons, 1992.

———. "Juan Bautista Peset y Vidal y las 'generaciones intermedias' del XIX español." *Medicina Española* 46 (1961): 186–203.

Loriga, Sabina. "The Plurality of the Past: Historical Time and the Rediscovery of Biography." In *The Biographical Turn: Lives in History,* ed. Hans Renders and J. Harmsa, 31–41. New York: Routledge, 2017.

Martín Araguz, Antonio. "Spanish Brain Science and Philosophy of Mind in the Time of Cervantes: Three Seminal Thinkers." In *Cervantes and the Early Modern Mind,* ed. Isabel Jaén and Julien Jacques Simon. New York: Routledge, 2022.

———, and Cristina Bustamante Martínez. "Examen de ingenios, de Juan Huarte de San Juan, y los albores de la neurobiología de la inteligencia en el Renacimiento español." *Revista de neurología* 38, no. 12 (2004): 1176–85.

———, C. Bustamente Martínez, and V. Fernández Armayor. "El suco nerveo sabuceano y los orígenes de la neuroquímica en el Renacimiento español." *Revista de Neurología* 36, no. 12 (June 2003): 1190–98.

Martykánová, Darina, and Víctor Manuel Núñez García. "Ciencia, patria y honor: los médicos e ingenieros y la masculinidad romántica en España (1820–1860)." *Studia historica. Historia contemporánea* 38 (2020): 45–75.

———. "Luces de España: las «ciencias útiles» durante el Trienio Constitucional." *Ayer: Revista de Historia Contemporánea* 127, no. 3 (June 17, 2022): 107–34.

McNeely, Ian F. *"Medicine on a Grand Scale": Rudolf Virchow, Liberalism, and the Public Health.* London: Wellcome Trust Centre for the History of Medicine, 2014.

Meister, Daniel R. "The Biographical Turn and the Case for Historical Biography." *History Compass* 16, no. 1 (2018). doi.org/10.1111/hic3.12436.

Miqueo, Consuelo. "Función de la prensa médica española en la difusión de la médecine physiologique (1820–1850)." *El Argonauta español. Revue bilingue, franco-espagnole, d'histoire moderne et contemporaine consacrée à l'étude de la presse espagnole de ses origines à nos jours (XVIIe–XXIe siècles)*, no. 8 (January 15, 2011). doi.org/10.4000/argonauta.83.

———, and Rosa Ballester, eds. "Dossier: Biografías médicas, una reflexión historiográfica." *Asclepio* 57, no. 1 (2005).

Molina Cantero, Camila. *Juan Huarte de San Juan y su Examen de ingenios para las ciencias. Exposición bibliográfica y documental con motivo del día del patrón de la Facultad de Psicología.* Granada: Gami Editorial, 2016. digibug.ugr.es.

Moreno Luzón, Javier, Ferran Archilés i Cardona, Fernando Molina Aparicio, and Sebastian Balfour. *Construir España: nacionalismo español y procesos de nacionalización.* Madrid: Centro de Estudios Políticos y Constitucionales, 2007.

———, and Xosé Manoel Núñez Seixas. *Los colores de la patria: símbolos nacionales en la España contemporánea.* Madrid: Tecnos, 2017.

Moro, José María. *Las epidemias de cólera en la Asturias del siglo XIX.* Oviedo: Servicio de Publicaciones de la Universidad de Oviedo, 2003.

Mounk, Yascha. "Italians Didn't Exactly Vote for Fascism." *The Atlantic,* September 26, 2022. www.theatlantic.com/ideas/archive/2022/09/italy-election-far-right-winner-giorgia-meloni-fascism/671556/.

Musolff, Andreas. "Political Metaphor and Bodies Politic." In *Discourse Approaches to Politics, Society and Culture,* ed. Urszula Okulska and Piotr Cap, 23–42. Amsterdam: John Benjamins Publishing Co., 2010.

Navarro Brotons, Víctor. "La polémica sobre la Inquisición y la ciencia en la España moderna. Consideraciones historiográficas y estado actual de la cuestión." In *La polemica europea sull'Inquisizione,* ed. Ugo Baldini, 123–44. Roma: Edizioni di storia e letteratura, 2015.

———, and William Eamon, eds. *Mas allá de la leyenda negra: España y la revolución científica = Beyond the Black Legend: Spain and the Scientific Revolution.* Valencia: Instituto de Historia de la Ciencia y Documentación López Piñero: Universitat de Valéncia: C.S.I.C., 2007.

Navarro, Jorge, and Jesús Gisbert. "La recepción del sensualismo en la España del siglo XIX: un estudio histórico." *Quaderns de Filosofia i Ciència* 8 (1985): 61–77.

Novella, Enric. *La ciencia del alma: locura y modernidad en la cultura española del siglo XIX.* Madrid: Iberoamericana, 2013.

———. *El discurso psicopatológico de la modernidad: ensayos de historia de la psiquiatría.* Madrid: Catarata, 2018.

———. "Medicina, antropología y orden moral en la España del siglo XIX." *Hispania. Revista Española de Historia* 70, no. 236 (2010): 709–36.

———. "La medicina de las pasiones en la España del siglo XIX." *Dynamis* 31, no. 2 (2011): 453–73.

————. "La política del yo: el espiritualismo psicológico en la cultura española de mediados del siglo XIX." *Asclepio* 62, no. 2 (December 30, 2010): 453–82.

Olmo, Ismael del. "La posesión diabólica en el Examen de ingenios para las sciencias (1575) de Juan Huarte de San Juan: Una paradoja." *Tiempos Modernos* 8, no. 33 (December 31, 2016): 70–101.

Pardo-Tomás, José, and Tomás Martínez Vidal. "Victims and Experts: Medical Practitioners and the Spanish Inquisition." In *Coping with Sickness: Medicine, Law and Human Rights. Historical Perspectives,* ed. John Woodward and Robert Jütte, 11–27. Sheffield, UK: European Association for the History of Medicine and Health Publications, 2000.

Payne, Stanley. *Spain: A Unique History.* Madison: University of Wisconsin Press, 2011.

Pérez Ledesma, Manuel, and María Sierra, eds. *Culturas políticas: Teoría e historia.* Zaragoza: Institución Fernando el Católico, 2010.

Pérez Vidal, Alejandro. *Bartolomé José Gallardo: Sátira, pensamiento y política.* Mérida: Editora Regional de Extremadura, 1999.

Peters, Edward. "Henry Charles Lea and the 'Abode of Monsters.'" In *The Spanish Inquisition and the Inquisitorial Mind,* ed. Alcalá, 577–608.

Pick, Daniel. *Faces of Degeneration: A European Disorder, c.1848–c.1918.* Cambridge, UK: Cambridge University Press, 1999.

Pimentel, Juan, and José Pardo-Tomás. "And yet we were modern. The paradoxes of Iberian science after the Grand Narratives." *History of Science; Special Issue: Iberian Science, Reflections and Studies* 55, no. 2 (2017): 133–47.

Plastina, Sandra. "Oliva Sabuco de Nantes and Her Nueva Filosofia: A New Philosophy of Human Nature and the Interaction between Mind and Body." *British Journal for the History of Philosophy* 27, no. 4 (2019): 738–52.

Porter, James I. "What Is 'Classical' about Classical Antiquity? Eight Propositions." *Arion* 13, no. 1 (2005): 27–61.

Porter, Roy. *Doctor of Society: Thomas Beddoes and the Sick Trade in Late-Enlightenment England.* New York: Routledge, 1992.

Pretel, Aurelio. "El enigma Sabuco: el parto de los montes." *Cultural Albacete* 12–13 (January 1, 2008): 10–26.

Ramón Fernández, Tomás. *La "década moderada" y la emergencia de la administración contemporánea.* Madrid: Iustel, 2021.

Ramos, Tomás. "La polémica hipocrática en la medicina española del siglo XIX." *Archivo iberoamericano de historia y de la medicina antropológica médica* 6 (1954): 115–61.

Read, Malcolm K. *Juan Huarte de San Juan.* Boston: Twayne Publishers, 1981.

Redondo, A. "La métaphore du corps de la république à travers le traité du médicine Jerónimo Merola (1587)." In *Le corps comme métaphore cans l'Espagne ces XVI et XVII siècles: du corps métaphorique aux métaphores corporelles,* 41–54. Paris: Publications de la Sorbonne, 1992.

Reed, Edward. *From Soul to Mind: The Emergence of Psychology from Erasmus Darwin to William James.* New Haven, CT: Yale University Press, 1997.

Renders, Hans. "Exceptions That Prove the Rule: Biography, Microhistory, and Marginals in Dutch Cities." In *Microhistory and the Picaresque Novel. A First Exploration into Commensurable Perspectives,* ed. Binne de Haan and Konstantin Mierau, 69–81. Newcastle upon Tyne: Cambridge Scholars Publishing, 2014.

———, and Binne De Haan. *Theoretical Discussions of Biography: Approaches from History, Microhistory and Life Writing.* Rev. ed. Leiden; Brill, 2014.

Rey González, Antonio M. "Clásicos de la psiquiatría del siglo XIX (IX): Juan Bautista Peset y Vidal (1821–1885)." *Revista de la Asociación Española de Neuropsiquiatría* 5, no. 12 (1985): 87–98.

Richardson, Alan. *British Romanticism and the Science of the Mind.* New York: Cambridge University Press, 2001.

Riera, J. "Matias Nieto y Serrano (1813–1902) y la medicina romántica." *Asclepio* 32 (1980): 367–81.

Rigoli, Juan. "The 'Novel of Medicine.'" In *Vitalism and the Scientific Image in Post-Enlightenment Life Science, 1800–2010,* ed. Sebastian Normandin and Charles T. Wolfe, 77–101. Heidelberg: Springer Netherlands, 2013.

Roca Barea, María Elvira. *Fracasología: España y sus élites: De los afrancesados a nuestros días.* Barcelona: Espasa, 2019.

Rohr, Isabelle. "Philosephardism and Antisemitism in Turn-of-the-Century Spain." *Historical Reflections/Réflexions Historiques* 31, no. 3 (Fall 2005): 373–92.

Romeo Mateo, María Cruz. "Lenguaje y política del nuevo liberalismo: Moderados y progresistas, 1834–1845." In *La política en el reinado de Isabel II,* ed. Isabel Burdiel, 37–62. Madrid: Marcial Pons, 1998.

———, and María Sierra. *Historia de las culturas políticas en España y América Latina. Vol. 2: La España liberal: 1833–1874.* Madrid: Marcial Pons Historia, 2014.

Ronzón, Elena. *Antropología y antropologías: Ideas para una historia crítica de la antropología española: el siglo XIX.* Oviedo: Pentalfa, 1991.

Rosa, Hartmut. *Resonance: A Sociology of Our Relationship to the World.* Medford, MA: Polity Press, 2019.

Rosenberg, Charles E. *Explaining Epidemics and Other Studies in the History of Medicine.* New York: Cambridge University Press, 1992.

Rubio Pobes, Coro. "Patria y nación." In *La creación de las culturas políticas modernas, 1808–1833,* vol. 1: *Historia de las culturas políticas en España y América Latina,* ed. Ángel Cabrera and Pro Ruiz, 97–125.

Ruggiero, Guido. "The Cooperation of Physicians and the State in the Control of Violence in Renaissance Venice." *Journal of the History of Medicine and Allied Sciences* 33, no. 2 (April 1978): 156–66.

Ruiz Torres, Pedro. "Modelos sociales del liberalismo español." In *Orígenes del liberalismo. Universidad, política, economía,* ed. Ricardo Robledo, Irene Castells, and María Cruz Romeo, 173–204. Salamanca: Universidad de Salamanca, 2003.

Rújula López, Pedro, and Manuel Chust Calero, eds. *El Trienio Liberal: Revolución e independencia.* Madrid: Los Libros de la Catarata, 2020.

Sánchez León, Pablo. "Introduction." In *Las jornadas de julio (de 1854): (una crónica anónima de "otro" 15M en el pasado ciudadano español)*, ed. Germán Labrador Méndez and Pablo Sánchez León. Madrid: Postmetropolis Editorial, 2018.

Sánchez Villa, Mario César. *Entre materia y espíritu: modernidad y enfermedad social en la España liberal (1833–1923)*. Madrid: Consejo Superior de Investigaciones Científicas, 2017.

Segarra, Josep Ramon. "La turbación de los tiempos: Ruptura temporal e historia en la construcción de las culturas políticas." In *La creación de las culturas políticas modernas, 1808–1833*, vol. 1: *Historia de las culturas políticas en España y América Latina*, ed. Ángel Cabrera and Pro Ruiz, 155–83.

Seoane Sobral, Mateo. *M. Seoane, la introducción en España del sistema sanitario liberal, 1791–1870*. Ed. José María López Piñero. Madrid: Servicio de Publicaciones, Ministerio de Sanidad y Consumo, 1984.

Serés, Guillermo. "Huarte de San Juan: de la 'naturaleza' a la 'política.'" *Criticón* 49 (1990): 77–90.

Shapin Steven. *A Social History of Truth: Civility and Science in Seventeenth-Century England*. Chicago: University of Chicago Press, 1994.

Shortland, Michael, and Richard R. Yeo. *Telling Lives in Science: Essays on Scientific Biography*. New York: Cambridge University Press, 1996.

Sierra, Maria. "La cultura politica en el estudio del liberalismo y sus conceptos de representación." In *Culturas políticas: teoría e historia*, ed. Pérez Ledesma and Sierra, 233–61.

———. "Política, romanticismo y masculinidad: Tassara (1817–1875)." *Historia y política: Ideas, procesos y movimientos sociales* 27 (2012): 203–26.

Sigurður G. Magnússon, and István M. Szijártó. *What Is Microhistory? Theory and Practice*. London: Routledge, Taylor & Francis Group, 2013.

Siraisi, Nancy G. *History, Medicine, and the Traditions of Renaissance Learning*. Ann Arbor: University of Michigan Press, 2007.

Sirinelli, Jean-François. "De la demeure à l'agora. Pour une histoire culturelle de politique." In *Axes et méthodes de l'histoire politique*. Paris: PUF, 1998.

Snell, Robert. *Portraits of the Insane: Theodore Gericault and the Subject of Psychotherapy*. London: Karnac Books, 2017.

Staum, Martin. "Cabanis and the Science of Man." *Journal of the History of the Behavioral Sciences* 10, no. 2 (1974): 135–43.

———. *Cabanis: Enlightenment and Medical Philosophy in the French Revolution*. Princeton, NJ: Princeton University Press, 1980.

Suárez Fernández, Constantino. *Escritores y artistas asturianos: índice bio-bibliográfico*. Ed. José María Martínez Cachero. Vol. 4. Madrid: Sáez impr., 1936.

Sumillera, Rocío G. "Political Medicine in Early Modern Spain, or How Physicians Counsel the King." *Sixteenth Century Journal* 51, no. 2 (2020): 419–42.

Torner, F. M. *Doña Oliva Sabuco de Nantes*. Madrid: M. Aguilar, 1935.

Torrecilla, Jesús. *España al revés: los mitos del pensamiento progresista (1790–1840)*. Madrid: Marcial Pons Historia, 2016.

Trim, Richard. *Metaphor and the Historical Evolution of Conceptual Mapping*. New York: Palgrave Macmillan, 2011.

Uzcanga Meinecke, Francisco. *¿Qué se debe a España? La polémica que dividió a la Europa de la Ilustración*. Madrid: Libros del K.O., 2021.

Valenzuela Calendario, José. "El espejismo del ejercicio libre. La ordenación de la asistencia médica en la España decimonónica." *Dynamis* 14 (1995): 296–304.

Vázquez García, Francisco. *La invención del racismo: Nacimiento de la biopolítica en España, 1600–1940*. Madrid: Akal, 2009.

Vicente-Pedraz, Miguel. "Cuerpo y política en la república original (1587), de Jerónimo Merola (A propósito de un caso de la metáfora organicista en el siglo de oro español)." *Andamios* 15, no. 36 (April 2018): 239–63.

Vidal, Fernando. *The Sciences of the Soul: The Early Modern Origins of Psychology*. Chicago: University of Chicago Press, 2011.

Villar Ortega, Helena. *Esclavos unidos: la otra cara del American Dream*. Madrid: Ediciones Akal, 2021.

Vintró, María C., and Mary Ellen Waithe. "¿Fue Oliva o fue Miguel? Reconsiderando el caso Sabuco." *Boletín del Instituto de Investigaciones Bibliográficas* 5, no. 1–2 (August 22, 2013). publicaciones.iib.unam.mx/index.php/boletin/article/view/646.

Waithe, Mary Ellen, and Maria Vintró. "Postumously Plagiarizing Oliva Sabuco: An Appeal to Catologuing Librarians." *Cataloguing and Classification Quarterly* 35, no. 3–4 (2003): 525–40.

Williams, Elizabeth A. *The Physical and the Moral: Anthropology, Physiology, and Philosophical Medicine in France, 1750–1850*. New York: Cambridge University Press, 1994.

Wolfe, Charles T. "The Animal Economy as Object and Program in Montpellier Vitalism." *Science in Context* 21, no. 4 (2008): 537–79.

———. "Expanded Mechanism and/or Structural Vitalism: Further Thoughts on the Animal Economy." In *Mechanism, Life and Mind in Modern Natural Philosophy*, ed. Charles T. Wolfe, Paolo Pecere, and Antonio Clericuzio. Cham: Springer International Publishing, 2022.

———. "Forms of Materialist Embodiment." In *Anatomy and the Organization of Knowledge, 1500–1850*, ed. Matthew Landers and Brian Muñoz, 129–44. London: Routledge, 2016.

Zavadil, Jeffery. "Anatomy of the Body Politic: Organic Metaphors in Ancient and Medieval Political Thought." PhD diss., Arizona State University, 2006.

Zozaya, María. "'Moral Revenge of the Crowd' in the 1854 Revolution in Madrid." *Bulletin for Spanish and Portuguese Historical Studies* 37, no. 1 (2012).

Zurita Aldeguer, Rafael. "El progresismo: Héroes e historia de la nación liberal." In *La España liberal: 1833–1874*, ed. Cruz Romeo and Sierra, vol. 2: 317–46.

Index